MEANING-FULLNESS

MEANING-FULLNESS
Developmental Psychotherapy and the Pursuit of Mental Health

Jan Resnick

With a foreword by

Nancy McWilliams

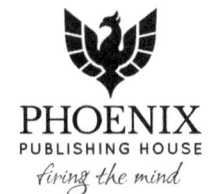

PHOENIX
PUBLISHING HOUSE
firing the mind

First published in 2023 by
Phoenix Publishing House Ltd
62 Bucknell Road
Bicester
Oxfordshire OX26 2DS

British Library Cataloguing in Publication Data

A C.I.P. for this book is available from the British Library

ISBN-13: 978-1-800131-33-0

Typeset by Medlar Publishing Solutions Pvt Ltd, India

www.firingthemind.com

This book is dedicated to the memory of

John M. Heaton

and

R. D. Laing

with respect, admiration, and love

My immeasurable debt of learning
can only be paid forward

"Step by step I progressed,
until I again became a human being."

Viktor Frankl in *Man's Search for Meaning*
on the time following his release
from the concentration camp (2014, p. 84)

Contents

Acknowledgements

There have been many influences on my development as a person and psychotherapist, and on the development of this book. I want to acknowledge general influences as well as specific people that have contributed, including:

My university education at Franconia College, New Hampshire, which was unusual and inspirational; the Guild of Psychotherapists (London) who gave me a clinical training and theoretical grounding in psychoanalytic psychotherapy, especially Christopher Bollas and Neville Symington; the Philadelphia Association (London) which delivered an advanced training and a post-phenomenological critique of psychoanalysis and supported my PhD, especially R. D. Laing, John M. Heaton, Francis Huxley, Hugh Crawford, Haya Oakley, Chris Oakley, Leon Redler, and Steve Gans.

My training analysis with Rosemary Gordon, then President of the Society of Analytical Psychologists (London).

The Collegium Phaenomenologicum (Perugia, Italy) for two summer schools with a focus on Martin Heidegger and Maurice Merleau-Ponty.

The Churchill Clinic (Perth, Western Australia)—as Director of Training for eighteen years I delivered over 2,000 seminars—itself an incredible learning experience. I acknowledge my faculty and students.

The national journal *Psychotherapy in Australia*, especially my friend and editor Liz Sheean, for twenty years of supporting my Commentary column in almost every issue.

The International Association for Relational Psychoanalysis and Psychotherapy for many conferences, workshops, colloquia, and publications that have been influential.

The Supervision Group of Developmental Paediatricians at the State Child Development Centre, Perth.

The Royal Australian/New Zealand College of Psychiatrists where I work with other psychotherapy supervisors.

The past thirty years of the Supervision Group attended by colleagues in counselling, psychology, psychotherapy, and psychoanalysis, for countless case discussions. And the many patients that have consulted me for psychotherapy over the course of my career. There is no greater learning than that gleaned from clinical experience where it has been my privilege to attend and work collaboratively in the most private spaces of the heart, mind, and soul.

I acknowledge those who have had an impact on this book:

Kate Pearce and the team at Phoenix Publishing House have improved this book and made the process of producing it enjoyable, notably unlike the experiences of some colleagues elsewhere.

The erudite Con Coroneos, who has been involved in the structure, writing style, content, and development of ideas. He has combed through most drafts of the manuscripts and helped to improve them. He has supported and encouraged me throughout and corrected many flaws and faults along the way, making this a much better book. I am grateful for our creative partnership.

Nancy McWilliams: for our friendship and for giving detailed feedback on the manuscript and many pertinent suggestions including related readings. Nancy edited the final draft in its entirety and made numerous suggestions.

Sue Lutton has read many drafts giving valuable perspectives; Samantha Kaiser made many useful comments and suggestions on two drafts; Ross Bolleter has made thoughtful contributions; Humphrey Bower gave valuable feedback; Jim Goodbourn also gave helpful feedback; Daniel Weber made useful comments; I appreciated remarks from Simon Byrne, John Wray, Sidrah Khan, Natasa Starcevich, Liz Sheean, Ros White, Marie-Laure Davenport, and Sally Richardson.

As this book is focused on early and subsequent childhood development, it feels important to acknowledge Sue Coleson, Cath Resnick, and my six children, Sean, Mischa, Lauren, Reece, Josh, and Gabriel, and three grandchildren, River, Beatrix and Odette—as parenting, co-parenting, and grandparenting are an invaluable education, undoubtedly my favourite roles. River is responsible for the painting on the jacket cover, done when she was four years old. Some of my adult children gave thoughtful reflections on the text especially Mischa Resnick, Gabriel Resnick, and Sean Resnick. Lauren Resnick assisted in the cover design. Lastly, my wife Cath Resnick has been a constant supporter of the all-consuming process of producing this book, as well as a fierce, but fair critic.

Foreword

Nancy McWilliams

It is my pleasure to introduce readers to the fertile mind of Jan Resnick, whom I met in the mid-1990s, when he invited me to Perth, Australia, to do a workshop for therapists in the psychotherapy training programme he had founded there. Over the years since that visit, he has come to be a trusted colleague and friend. Dr Resnick has a prodigious intellect and a big heart; to me, he exemplifies the best in the psychoanalytic clinical tradition. In this foreword, I introduce readers to his sensibility and his knack for passing on psychoanalytic wisdom.

Whatever your level of sophistication about psychotherapy, you will learn a lot from this book and, even better, you can expect to enjoy reading it. Written without jargon, self-inflation, or pretension, it explores—in accessible and even entertaining language—ideas that often come across as dense and complicated. Clinical vignettes, offered candidly and with the author's description of his own emotional involvement in the patient's story as it unfolds in each session, illuminate the developmental concepts that have inspired the book.

There was a time when Dr Resnick's phrase "developmental psychotherapy" would not have been necessary to specify what a mental health professional does in the role of therapist. But the social construction of psychotherapy itself has changed over the last couple of decades. Up until fairly recently, therapy was widely understood, in both professional and nonprofessional cultures, as in its essence a maturational process that requires a relationship of sufficient emotional safety to invite the evolving expression, exploration, and eventual transcendence of painful and shameful aspects of self. In recent times, the term "psychotherapy" has been used much more promiscuously to designate any intervention designed to make someone feel better or provide a quick fix for the person's most disabling symptoms.

Our original construct of psychotherapy, rooted in evolving theory, accumulated clinical experience, and research (on personality, psychological development, affect, defence, therapy process, and other areas relevant to treatment) assumed that clinicians pay attention to the ways each person's emotional maturation got somehow stalled or misdirected, and that we work with clients collaboratively to reduce impediments to the resumption of their growth. In other words, we help people who have been knocked off the rails by stressful or traumatic life experiences to get back on track. We foster a process in which they can find the courage to change what can be changed and to grieve and move on from what cannot be changed. In this book, one witnesses Dr Resnick's appreciation not only of his patients' developmental arrests but also their developmental accomplishments, often achieved in the face of formidable obstacles. He understands that their ways of being in the world and with themselves represent the best adaptation they could make to their developmental challenges. Together, he and his clients build on their health-seeking propensities to meet life's current challenges.

In recent years, for numerous intersecting reasons that amount to a perfect storm, psychotherapy has been conceptualised much less developmentally. This happened originally in the United States but quickly spread to Dr Resnick's Australia and other countries. Assumptions about a complex and ultimately unpredictable interactive process have devolved into the prototype of a knowledgeable expert applying proven technical procedures that reduce measurable symptoms. The causes of this desiccation of what most therapists consider their sacred calling are complex and multifarious, but they surely include the following: (1) the interests of pharmaceutical companies in framing psychological treatments in terms of simple symptom-reduction (so that they can market drugs for those symptoms); (2) the interests of insurance companies and government bureaucrats in believing that meaningful change can happen much faster than is usually realistic (so that their financial outlays are reduced); (3) the interests of some academic researchers, especially those who conduct time-limited studies of manualised interventions.

With respect to the last influence, we have seen a limited research paradigm replace a complex clinical one. I have rarely met a therapist who thinks research is unimportant; most of us believe that treatment should be based not only on what admired mentors have recommended but also on what science has demonstrated. But a commitment to *basing* psychotherapy on empirical studies is a very different matter from assuming that the therapy process itself should *resemble* a certain kind of limited outcome research. The philosophers whose work influenced Dr Resnick's writing might refer to the latter as a category error, the intrusion of a paradigm that serves one discipline or objective into an area it doesn't fit.

In much outcome research, one selects patient volunteers without comorbidities, takes measures of symptoms at the onset of the study, uses graduate students as the therapists, requires them to follow manuals, delimits the length of the study, and assesses improvement by changes in measured symptoms. In actual practice, in contrast, most therapists do not screen patients to select those with one DSM disorder not comorbid with any other, or take baseline measurements or manualise what we do. Where possible, we leave length of treatment up to the patient, and we judge improvement in terms of overall life satisfactions rather than specific symptom reduction. Research on patient satisfaction suggests that when people feel their therapist is following a protocol rather than responding to their individuality, they tend to devalue the therapy.

This conflation between concepts that apply to research and concepts that characterise psychotherapy may derive from the fact that most contemporary academic psychologists, even those who teach abnormal or clinical psychology, have scant experience of psychotherapy as it happens outside the psychology laboratory. It would probably amount to professional suicide for a contemporary academic to become immersed in clinical training at the expense of time to pursue grants and conduct research. And realistically, it has become so difficult in universities to attain tenure and/or promotion that professors understandably prefer their curriculum vitae to show a long list of publications of short studies rather than a short list of in-depth research on topics of the complexity seen in actual clinical practice. In addition, it is no longer common for academic psychologists to have had their own therapy. Given the demands on their time, they may not see the point of it unless they are suffering from incapacitating symptoms.

One result of changes in university culture is that academic psychologists often misunderstand and devalue psychotherapists—they resent our not always practising in line with how they interpret their research, and they tend to misperceive the nature of our work. Because the "patients" they study are often student volunteers who claim to have one disorder "not comorbid with anything else", their experience can be quite distant from working with the complexly troubled people that clinicians typically see. (I can't remember the last time I saw a patient with a symptomatic problem that was unrelated to a personality issue, a post-traumatic condition, a substance-use problem, a situational challenge, or some other complication). As a result of their relative isolation from clinical work, academic psychologists often misunderstand our theories and how we apply them to practice. Most contemporary academics, for example, seem to think that today's psychoanalysts are ideologically wedded to Freud's earliest ideas—perhaps because that may be all they have read about the long psychoanalytic clinical tradition.

Some of this revision of our shared understanding of the nature of therapy reflects from long-ago decisions to construe psychological problems as categorical and descriptive diagnoses rather than as dimensional and inferential problems in living. By categorical, I mean that one either has or does not have a disorder, in contrast to the dimensional assumption that psychopathology is largely a matter of the *degree* to which a particular mental tendency, one with which many of us can identify, is causing trouble. By descriptive, I mean that what is externally observable or readily measurable is preferred to inferences about the *meaning* of symptoms. In the DSM, there is no concept of mental health, only descriptions of deviations from it. In specifying all the "disorders" that can arise in individuals, it lacks a focus on the origins of common difficulties in normal developmental processes that become somehow undermined or traumatically interrupted.

It is in this area that Dr Resnick's book is most passionate and critical. His distress about what has happened to his beloved profession is doubtless why he foregrounded meaning in the title. He insists, like any psychoanalytic therapist and most therapists of other orientations as well, that symptoms have meaning. Two people with identical DSM diagnoses of depression can have significantly different subjective experiences: one woman's low mood expresses her deep belief that she is internally corrupt, evil, and guilty, while another's reflects an internal world that is empty, lonely, and meaningless. Individuals with identical anxiety symptoms can feel radically different subjectively: one man is terrified of being destroyed; another dreads abandonment; another fears criticism; another expects a childhood sexual trauma to recur at any moment; another feels a sexual temptation and fears he will behave contrary to his moral beliefs. It is the therapist's job not simply to get rid of the depression or anxiety but to understand the symptom and address the psychology that gave rise to it. If, in general medicine, doctors classified physical suffering on the basis of what is externally observable and measurable (for example, "fever disorders", "skin rash disorders", and "limp disorders") and defined good medical care as the reduction of those symptoms without concern for their causes, we would be alarmed. But in the field of psychotherapy, we seem all too willing to accept this insult to common sense.

Every person is unique. Few therapists with any clinical experience expect to understand any client's mental suffering from lists of present-versus-absent diagnostic criteria. In fact, we don't expect *ever* to understand any client completely, even if we can comprehend enough of the person's story to help the narrative to change over time. A profound respect for each individual's capacity to chart an idiosyncratic course towards loving better, working better, and playing better underlies all our clinical work. Changes in these directions require the nourishing of a sense of self-respect and personal agency, qualities that are often absent or damaged in clients when they begin treatment. Everyone's timetable for accomplishing meaningful change is different and not predictable at the beginning of a therapeutic relationship. Each person's way of formulating and resolving their problems has to be discovered, not prescribed.

As a Winnicott scholar, Dr Resnick is keenly interested in the impoverishment of play. In fact, the playfulness of his writing style itself exemplifies what it describes. So many of our current patients are unable to play; some of them are unacquainted with even the idea of playfulness as a core part of health and growth. His book takes readers thoughtfully through Winnicott's thinking about play as the basis for creativity and the development of the capacity for meaning. Not only does an ability to play ultimately soften life's hard knocks, but we also know now empirically that all young mammals have a strong need for play and that without it, certain other mental capacities fail to develop. We should be paying attention to these findings.

With the current, well-documented explosion of mental health problems, especially in young people, including increases in serious mental illness, despair, and suicide that have accompanied the Covid-19 pandemic and will doubtless persist in its aftermath, it is vitally important that we not rely on a "psychotherapy" defined by the interests of businesspeople and bureaucrats who want us to apply formulas and check boxes. Therapists in this moment have a pressing obligation to help people restore their capacity to play. We should be bearing meaningful witness to all instances of suffering, whether or not the DSM captures that suffering in the definition of a "disorder" category. We should be able to offer help to those whom the recent plague has sidelined or isolated or bereaved or prevented from moving through the maturational milestones and rites of passage they had every reason to see as in their immediate future before the virus upended their expectations. It is hard enough to attain a sense of confident adulthood in a mass culture, in which one inevitably feels profoundly insignificant, without the ordeals created by the pandemic and all its attendant uncertainty, controversy, and polarisation.

This book is in the tradition of psychoanalytic phenomenology that seeks to understand rather than predict and control. It belongs to the hypothesis-generating rather than the hypothesis-testing tradition in science, in which the observer cannot claim separation from what is observed. Influenced by R. D. Laing, John M. Heaton, D. W. Winnicott, and others loosely affiliated with the British "Middle Group" of object-relations theorists, Jan Resnick commits to a subjective understanding of suffering and to the search for meaning as he shares the insights he has gleaned over a career that spans decades of working with widely diverse clients.

Meaning-Fullness is a pun, an expression of Winnicottian play, a serious exploration of the deeper meaning of words, and most meaning-full to me, a *cri de coeur* for a field that Dr Resnick loves, which he fears is being slowly destroyed by commercial, bureaucratic, paint-by-numbers notions of "psychotherapy". The writing flows, with a distinctive personal style marked by wit, self-irony, passion, and compassion. You may not agree with everything Dr Resnick says, but you will be stimulated by engaging with his mind, and you will learn a lot about what psychotherapy looks like in the hands of a wise elder.

Preface

Meaning-fullness is fullness of meaning: when you *feel* full, there is nothing missing from your experience of living. To understand this properly, first consider the opposite: the absence of meaning-fullness brings a sense of emptiness and nameless dread. In his landmark book *Man's Search for Meaning*, Viktor Frankl calls this "the existential vacuum". He says the feeling of meaninglessness arises when people have enough to live by, but nothing to live for:

> they have the means but not the meaning. (2014, p. 132)

These days, more and more people have neither. Ordinary living has become more expensive and it's getting worse. Without doubt, financial stress and pressure, and consequent busyness, leaves little room for questions of the meaning of living. But it isn't only that; there are a range of underlying reasons. Over more than forty years of psychotherapy practice, I have found the existential vacuum is a dominant feature of mental disorders and other psychological conditions. It does not feature in the DSM or bio-medical approaches.

My purpose in this book is to show why current mental health practices are falling short in the ever-growing need for effective responses to the epidemic of mental unwellness. The critique of current practices is only to put in context an alternative view of how to understand mental disorders differently from the prevailing medical and psychology perspectives and to offer an alternative vision of therapy that makes a meaningful difference.

This book places the existential vacuum in the forefront of the undergirding influences of mental unwellness in the endeavour to address the question: *What makes life worth living?* It is a question that is absent from most current mental health approaches that view psychological disorders as a medical pathology, a radical mistake.

This question invites exploration of some themes that Winnicott developed, most notably in his last published work *Playing and Reality* (1971). I elaborate his ideas on play and creativity, develop them further, and introduce the essential role of "language" in understanding and treating mental/emotional suffering.

A "developmental psychotherapy", as I am calling it, is one that takes the above themes into account in the service both of relieving mental suffering and promoting emotional and personal growth. The glib memes of social media on low self-esteem, forgiveness, gratitude, and acceptance hold traces of wisdom but rarely meet the profound needs of those in mental/emotional pain. A therapeutic process built on recognition, understanding, and an evolving professional relationship creates conditions for development, while addressing the painful issues that matter. I have set out to show how this can be done in the hope that mental health professionals reconsider their underlying suppositions and the current practices built on them.

A few practical points about the text: I use the terms "patient" and "client" interchangeably. I use the plural "they" or "them" grammatically incorrectly instead of using he and she or her and him, to avoid limiting, binary, gender stereotypes.

Lastly, I've tried to make the text readable, though it may be difficult in parts. If you find it too difficult, don't get bogged down. Better to skip over those passages and just move on. The book is written for people at different levels of understanding and experience in the mental health field but is not exclusively for mental health professionals. This work should be of value to anyone concerned with issues of mental health and well-being, personal development, and creating a meaning-full way of living.

Jan Resnick
Perth, Western Australia

Making your life worth living

What makes life worth living? I raise this question because I believe it is central to creating a sound foundation for mental health. For some, this question never arises. For others, it is so elusive as to be a constant mystery, or a source of puzzlement, disturbance, grief, and a drive to search for an answer.

The way the question is put expresses a sense that life *should* have a worth, it should *mean something*. Where does this "worth" come from? How does it arise? And what does it mean for mental health if there is no sense of worth in living?

As noted in the Preface, Viktor Frankl used the term "the existential vacuum" to describe how emptiness produces a sense of a life *not* worth living. Well before Frankl, Carl Jung said:

> About a third of my cases are suffering from no clinically definable neurosis, but from the senselessness and emptiness of their lives. This can be defined as the general neurosis of our times. (1933, p. 61)

Both Frankl and Jung saw the consequences of the existential vacuum that was growing to epidemic proportions. We are there now, living in that epidemic, made worse by the Covid-19 pandemic. It is one of the most urgent and pervasive socio-cultural issues of our time. Currently, many social ills are, to some extent, a direct expression of it. They include poverty, unemployment, violence and crime, relationship breakdown, addictions and substance abuse, self-harm, and a great deal of mental illness and psychosomatic disorders. Add worsening suicide statistics to the mix and you have a society in crisis.

As a therapist, I encounter this crisis constantly. I am struck by how many patients have difficulty finding or making meaning anywhere in their lives and how this relates to anxiety, depression, and other mental health conditions. Again, helping them with this is not easy but there is enormous merit in an approach that recognises the significance of *meaning*.

Meaning is a huge subject about which much has been written. My approach is inspired by the work of Donald Winnicott, R. D. Laing, and John M. Heaton, with a focus upon Winnicott's last published work *Playing and Reality* (1971). This book stands out for me as one of the most important in the corpus of psychoanalytic literature. Why? Partly because it raises the question of what makes life worth living as central to the therapeutic endeavour.

Winnicott shows how the capacity for meaning-making originates for babies and young children and, by extension, how meaning can be found or made by adults. Many people do raise the question: *Is anything inherently meaningful?* Some wake up at a certain point and wonder *Why am I doing this? I'm not happy. Nothing means that much to me. Why am I living like this? Why am I living?* Such questions arise early for some and much later for others—though they can arise at any time.

Winnicott is important to me for personal reasons, too. Winnicott supervised R. D. Laing when Laing trained as a psychoanalyst. And Laing supervised me when I trained as a psycho-therapist. Laing became the most widely read psychiatrist/psychoanalyst in the world from the 1960s, through the 1980s, and left an indelible mark on how we understand and work with mental unwellness. Arguably, the Laingian shift from the analysis of a patient's mind to a focus on the therapeutic relationship spawned what later became the contemporary movement of relational psychoanalysis and psychotherapy. Now, despite vast differences in practice modalities, mental health professionals usually agree on the centrality of the professional relationship—as countless empirical studies now show—and its essential role as an agent of healing and growth.

I worked with John Heaton over sixteen years and never tired of engaging in often dense philosophical texts and considering their application to the clinical work of psychotherapy. In his later work, Heaton published important works on Wittgenstein, the role of language, and psychotherapy. Heaton's influence on my thinking and practice is immeasurable. Philosophy is the love of wisdom and nowhere is wisdom needed more than now to meet the growing epidemic of mental suffering.

I never met Winnicott, but I feel he is in my DNA, professionally speaking. DNA is the molecule that carries genetic instruction for growth, development, and the functioning of all living organisms; this describes how I view my professional lineage. It is no guarantee of anything, certainly not of being a "good therapist" or knowing what I'm talking about; I just like the idea. Of course, literal DNA does not necessarily guarantee how any individual's life turns out either, what may be achieved, or what your destiny turns out to be. Important as it is, there is more to life than biology. Your life depends on what you make it, at least in part, and on what it makes you.

Your life is what you make it, and what it makes you.

The problem of meaninglessness can at least be mitigated. Winnicott's ideas, somewhat obscure in the original, are profoundly helpful when rendered more intelligible and elaborated.

After completing the manuscript of *Meaning-fullness*, I mentioned this project to a friend and colleague in London. She responded: "I studied *Playing and Reality* chapter by chapter with Winnicott's wife Clare Winnicott who said Donald was unhappy with the language he had employed there, he felt he was still pandering too much to Melanie Klein." I indulged in the fantasy that Donald Winnicott was endorsing this enterprise, albeit posthumously.

The above led me to a now famous letter from Winnicott to Melanie Klein in which he acknowledges annoying her by stating his own ideas in his own way and confronts her by saying that he will not stifle his own creative gesture because of her agenda to foreclose language in psychoanalytic meetings to a closed theoretical system, namely her own.

> This language must, however, be kept alive as there is nothing worse than a dead language.
> (Winnicott in Newman, 1995, p. 8)

This comment speaks to the endeavour here. By engaging critically with his thinking in *Playing and Reality*, and unpacking the ideas in clear, jargon-free, language, we can relate Winnicott's views to the contemporary scene with respect to mental health and, more generally, living.

The aim of our journey in this book is to light a path for making your life worth living through showing how to live meaningfully and how to get meaningful help when you can't find your way or find you're stumbling through the darkness—or worse, becoming mentally unwell.

My relationship to psychoanalysis

Winnicott started his professional life as a paediatrician and his own development took him to psychoanalysis. Early on, he was supervised by Melanie Klein and identified as a Freudian, though his work is an implicit criticism and departure from the thinking of Freud and of Klein. Both were concerned with unconscious forces, instincts, and phantasy (the *ph* refers to the unconscious). Winnicott, far from opposed to those issues, was more focused on child development and the influence of *actual* experience upon later development and, specifically, the sort of mental health conditions brought for treatment.

Laing started his professional life as a psychiatrist and then became a psychoanalyst. His ideas shifted the focus of therapy from the analysis of an individual mind to a foregrounding of the interpersonal professional relationship and how various mental disorders manifest themselves within the consulting situation. He was acutely aware of confusions in communications, meta-communications, and miscommunications as well as the over-medicalisation of psychopathology and its treatments. He regarded both the historical context of childhood experience and family dynamics, and the present context as indispensable for an understanding of mental unwellness.

The history of psychoanalysis later evolves through the work of Stephen A. Mitchell and colleagues into a movement called relational psychoanalysis and psychotherapy that has grown from its New-York-centric origins to an international group that has produced a significant body of literature on theory and practice.

In particular, the work of Donnel B. Stern (2003, 2010, 2019) traverses a somewhat similar territory as *Meaning-Fullness* does here, albeit with important differences. Over a trilogy of erudite works, he has developed a theory of mind that departs from the former psychoanalytic understanding of the unconscious. Instead of "the unconscious" as a noun that implies a container of unknown forces and meanings, for Stern meaning emerges through experience not-yet-formulated into an articulable language and hence remains unsymbolised. The professional relationship and therapy process elicits a ripening of the material, that becomes formed through the process of symbolisation. (This will be unpacked in greater detail later.)

Stern could also be called a philosophical hermeneuticist (focused on interpretation) and constructivist (how meaning is constructed)—and these have their own traditions for those interested—unlike the work of Jacques Lacan who draws more from structural linguistics and represents a more Euro-centric intellectual tradition. Both understand language to be the source of *all meaningfulness in human life* (Stern, 2019, p. 31)—a position shared here.

One essential difference is that I see psychotherapy as a craft, essentially a practice, that benefits from an emphasis upon ordinary human understanding and without a heavy reliance upon theory, such as psychoanalytic theory. To be fair, there are elements of psychoanalytic theory in this text, and one of the defining principles of the relational movement is precisely an aversion to excessive and dogmatic adherence to theory. For psychotherapy, it is better to resist theoretical identifications. My primary identification is as a clinician, a therapist. Accordingly, I am not a Freudian, Jungian, Winnicottian, Laingian, Sternian, logotherapist, or anything ending in *ian*.

I have tried to present a view of psychotherapy that is accessible, avoiding getting bogged down in a rarefied, intellectual discourse, while still being informed by philosophy—especially phenomenology and existentialism—and the collective clinical wisdom of psychoanalysis and psychotherapy. The aim is to make psychotherapy more readily understandable and a more effective response to the mental health crisis of our time.

The structure of the book

The book is in four parts.

Part I critiques the current state of mainstream mental health attitudes and approaches and their relationship to empirical research using randomised controlled trials of techniques applied to specific "disorders" as the undergirding source of knowledge. I discuss how such terms as "evidence", "science", and "research" have been bastardised in the service of the self-interest of some mental health professions and that of other corporate agendas. This is intended to contextualise the subsequent discussion of meaning and its relationship to mental health, and early childhood development as the original source of capacities for meaning-making.

Part I continues with a discussion of the existential vacuum illustrated through vignettes extracted from a case of psychotherapy. I go on to explore how the capacity to make meaning originates in early childhood experience. A discussion of language follows, illustrating how children become initiated into using language and come to express their sense of meaning. Initiation into language is no less an initiation into the local culture of the family in which a child grows, and by extension the broader community and, ultimately, global culture. The implications for a discussion of meaning in adult experience are profound and contribute to a foundation for mental health.

Part II focuses on play and creativity: the role of play in early childhood development and its value for the development of capacities for creativity in a broader sense. Meaning has to be found or made, and both require a capacity for creativity, a term employed luxuriously throughout. What is it? My use of "creativity" here refers to the formation of something new and valuable. The process is both internal (that is, mental), and external or practical. This includes gestation: something that cannot be seen yet involves growth and development. When it comes to therapy, creativity refers to a person's evolution into a more authentic sense of self, the formation of identity in the sense of the total personality. In this context, Winnicott uses the term "creativity" as a colouring of a person's "whole attitude to external reality" (1971, p. 65).

Part III extends the ideas of Parts I and II. It includes a critique of Winnicott and a further elaboration of his ideas. This leads to a philosophical analysis of the function of play with reference to the work of Hans-Georg Gadamer in his landmark book *Truth and Method*. Then, the importance of the professional relationship in developmental psychotherapy is illustrated through clinical examples.

Part IV synthesises and integrates the many ideas covered in the previous parts through a long clinical case that has challenged me for many years. I set out to demonstrate why spending time on one case over many years of a *developmental psychotherapy* works better than the quick-fix attitudes of the manualised approaches, now sometimes called "therapy". The whole book points in a different direction: how mental health therapies could be more effective and lasting.

* * *

While psychotherapy admittedly can take a long time, there is a false economy in treating people quickly, imagining them "better", only to see them return a short while later. This becomes a pattern that repeats, as many mental health professionals testify. I have heard countless accounts of the revolving door of mental health treatments for patients with files like encyclopaedias. This circularity could be called *a misery-go-round* and constitutes the epidemic of mental ill-health.

A developmental psychotherapy promotes finding and creating meaning through a certain quality of professional relationship, a relationship that simultaneously draws you out of yourself and puts you more in touch with yourself. Indeed, it is through relationship that meaning comes into being in the first place—whether with objects, activities, or another person, or any combination. I will show how this approach applies to specific mental health conditions such as anxiety and depression. When I speak of a developmental psychotherapy, it is with adults in mind and as distinct from what has been termed "Dyadic Developmental Psychotherapy"[1] which focuses on children with emotional disorders, complex trauma, and attachment issues. There, the dyad (the twosome) is the therapist and child-patient, whereas my work is primarily, though not exclusively, with adults.

At the same time, this book integrates early childhood experience, adult experience, and psychotherapy experience, moving fluidly through these domains. Each has a reference and a relevance to the other. Childhood experience is formative and defining for adult experience, expressed in therapy as memories or re-enactments. Adult experience affects how you remember and regard childhood experience; the actuality of what happened to you in the past cannot change, though how you have been affected by it *can*. In turn, psychotherapeutic experience informs adult experience, ultimately changing the way you experience yourself and what happens in your life. *The way you experience* is the basis of everything. What you make of what happens and how it affects you is the focus of a developmental psychotherapy.

When worked at, therapy engenders an enhanced capacity to find and create meaning. If that hasn't happened *early*, or early enough, it may not be too late. It still needs to happen later. Further development requires work. And the question of what makes life worth living is answered in a way personal to you. It's not the same for everyone but every person who can work in psychotherapy can build their capacity for meaning-fullness—it is an inborn potential—requiring development at the earliest possible opportunity to achieve a life worth living.

---

[1] DDP is attributed to Arthur Becker-Weidman and Daniel Hughes and is largely based on Bowlby's attachment theory though it combines other approaches in its treatment methods. There is some overlap as DDP is influenced by thinkers such as Daniel Stern and Alan Schore, as am I.

Part I

Meaning and meaninglessness

CHAPTER 1

The epidemic crisis of mental health

As far as we can discern,
the sole purpose of human existence
is to kindle a light of meaning
in the darkness of mere being.
C. G. Jung

It is becoming socially acceptable to admit to struggling mentally. The fears, anxieties, and terrible losses of the Covid-19 pandemic have contributed to the recognition of a crisis in mental health. Across the range of disorders and diagnoses, you can let others know you are in emotional pain, mental conflict, or distress, have such a low mood you cannot get out of bed, are too anxious or self-conscious to function socially or, in a word, can't cope.

As a therapist, I am deeply aware of this crisis. A common theme patients bring to the consulting room is a feeling of emptiness or purposelessness. Life has no meaning. *I don't know what I want and even if I did, I have no motivation to do anything, anyway.* There are the elusive questions of *Where do I belong?* and *Which direction to point in?* Alienation is rife. So is loneliness and the feeling of isolation. And with that, there is also the persistent dilemma of how to establish a good relationship, or how to make one work in the modern world.

The New York Times (Tavernise, 2016) reported that suicide rates in the United States had surged to their highest level in thirty years. A US federal data analysis reported increases in every age group except those over age seventy-five. (That surprised me.) The rate of increase doubled from 2006 on! There was a notably sharp increase in suicide amongst thirty-five to sixty-four-year-olds—the prime of life!

Earlier, a TED talk by Tom Insel (2013), then director of the US National Institute of Mental Health, provided more shocking statistics:

- One in five people will have a mental disorder or neuropsychiatric syndrome in their lifetime.
- One in twenty people are disabled by a mental illness, thirty per cent of which arise from a mental disorder.
- Of those suffering from a mental disorder, fifty per cent will have onset by age fourteen and seventy-five per cent will have onset by twenty-four.
- Ninety per cent of suicides are related to a mental disorder, that is, an average of 38,000 people every year, about one every fifteen minutes. In the year of his talk, 2013, 47,000 would die, more than from breast cancer.
- Suicide is the third most common cause of death for those aged fifteen to twenty-five, twice as common as homicide, and more common than traffic fatalities.

Such statistics are but a snapshot of a particular time and place. Suicide statistics vary and are contentious. Some say there are fewer suicides than before. Today, I hear more suicidal ideation than ever before, and not least from my youngest teenage patients.

Insel said we have been seeing mental disorders as either a disease of the mind or a behavioural disorder and this has been a terrible impediment to improving treatment outcomes. I agree. Then, he argues for a new understanding of mental disorders as brain disorders. Studying cognition or behaviour is simplistic and reductionistic compared with studying the surreal complexity of the organ of the brain, a massively complicated machine for an extraordinary amount of information processing.

I cringe at his language. Although accurate in some ways, I find it dehumanising and problematic. Advances in the understanding of the brain, in neuroscience and psychobiology, have made useful contributions to the understanding of mental disorders. Already, there are methods of early detection of brain changes that pre-date observable behaviour changes by a decade or more. Let's stop and think for a moment though: how will bio-medicine "treat" your brain to effect improvements in your mental health?

Obviously, psychoactive and neuroleptic medications are and will be employed. Psychosurgery and electroshock have been used already for quite some time. To what extent do medical scientists and then mental health practitioners *really* know what they're doing by interfering with the 100 billion neurons and 100 trillion synapses that compose this "machinery of surreal complexity"? I would feel very cautious indeed about allowing anyone to interfere with my brain, especially if they regard it as a machine or information-processing computer, and especially at a time when I am most vulnerable. Any consideration of history, context, primary relationships, life events, or personal experience of the world have gone out the window.

What is more, changes in the brain are not necessarily the causes of a mental disorder—a critical point that is frequently lost in the discussion of understanding mental illness as a brain disorder. When we identify a change in the brain, we identify a potential correlation with a change in personality, in mood, in your sense of yourself or your perceptions, and then often later, in behaviour. Could changes in your mental state cause changes in your brain chemistry or even structure? Maybe, but *correlation is not causation*—a point often overlooked in the purely bio-medical perspective. For me, this has much to do with the ineffectiveness of mainstream mental health practices and a culture overrun with mental unwellness and far too many suicides.

The idea of rewiring brains has become increasingly popular, new therapies are being developed based on this idea. For acquired brain injuries in which we can identify with some confidence that changes in the brain have affected mental functioning and personality, then the techniques of rewiring, re-programming, and re-learning or new learning often through the body are invaluable.[2]

For the one in five people with mental disorders, so-called re-wiring—or, more accurately, the creation of new neuronal pathways in the brain—occurs through new experiences. This is what we have been doing in psychotherapy since Freud launched psychoanalytic therapy over one hundred years ago. Well before Freud, and in less formal ways, psychotherapy can lay equal claim to being the oldest profession. Science has helped us understand better why it works from a physiological point of view,[3] but psychotherapists don't tend to think of therapy in terms of re-wiring. We are working with people, not robots. It makes a difference!

Whether you are suffering from a clearly defined diagnosable mental disorder or plagued by existential questions of meaning—*What is my life for?*—or even the more basic ontological questions of identity: *Who am I? Am I real?*—how do you get help?

Almost every person that consults me as a psychotherapist has been to multiple mental health professionals and not been helped. A few have been helped a little. Some have suffered harm: patients are left riled, annoyed, frustrated, angry, confused, disturbed, or feel *help* has been harmful. This disturbs me. Maybe the ones that have been helped never need to consult me? (I'm not implying that I have helped every patient.)

How can we create a meaningful response to the existential questions so pervasive in contemporary culture—a meaningful response to meaninglessness? How to fill the emptiness? How to find your way? How to change what needs to be changed, adjust where you must, and learn to live-with what defies alteration? How to know the difference? Where to receive guidance from those with experience and wisdom? And how to work things out for yourself where no one can guide or instruct you? Questions like: *What are my values? What do I really want? What is my direction? Who matters to me and to whom do I matter? What to do?* These are the fundamental questions that define and determine the transition from being-a-child to

---

[2] See the amazing work of Norman Doidge, for example, such as *The Brain that Changes Itself* and *The Brain's Way of Healing*.

[3] See Susan C. Vaughan (2019). *The Talking Cure: The Science Behind Psychotherapy* for a discussion on how talking therapy can affect changes in neuronal pathways in the brain. This is still correlation and not necessarily causation.

being-an-adult. Development is a transitional process and fraught with issues, feelings, confusions, and conflicts. There is much to work out and work through. Your mental health depends on the outcome.

Yet, this is not about measurable *outcomes*, a word so often synonymous with the short-term, quick-fix approaches that give the illusion of improvement on the questionnaires and surveys in such common use. They prove nothing. Typically, they are short cuts but why take a short cut when it's the journey that matters. Mental health and unwellness defy measure; the metrics are misleading, and largely function to reassure professionals that their simplistic efforts in the face of hugely complex, often long-standing issues, have been effective. Generalities about mental disorders only blind professionals to the most significant particulars that are unavoidably personal to every individual seeking help. The devil really is in the detail. Patients typically feel "missed" when manualised approaches are applied as if one size could ever fit all.

When it comes to mental unwellness, what is needed is a process that takes account of the present situation in the context of developmental and historical issues and the broader existential and metaphysical ones. When my patients feel better, the crisis that brought them abates, they find relief from suffering, and, better still, feel they've grown through the process of therapy. It is invariably the process generated through spending sufficient time on their issues that makes the difference. Professional relationships become increasingly therapeutic over time (as "epistemic trust"[4] grows) (Fonagy, Luyten, Allison, & Campbell, 2019).

Too many mental health practices have moved away from giving time and attention, cultivating rapport and empathic understanding, and developing insight into the meaning of experience and behaviour. In the service of faster outcomes, more lasting outcomes seem to have declined. The promotion of manualised treatments in psychology and more effective, targeted medications in psychiatry have generated the illusion that mainstream mental health approaches are winning the battle against mental ill health. The *evidence*[5] suggests otherwise, and I am afraid we are losing the war.

> If this is the future, we are pointing in the wrong direction.

More and more people have mental health issues, and they are taking medications and attending short-term psychology practices. In the Western world, as a culture, we are getting more

---

[4] Defined as openness to receiving social knowledge—in this context: learning from the therapist and therapy process.

[5] There are many sources for this assertion: see the National Institute for Mental Health—https://www.nimh.nih.gov/health/statistics/mental-illness.shtml or in Australia Beyond Blue—https://www.beyondblue.org.au/media/statistics. The statistics are alarming.

unwell despite the self-promoting assertions of psychology and psychiatry. Self-deception is rife in the mental health world; whole professions can be disordered, too.

Meanwhile, existential and metaphysical questions about the meaning of living have dropped off the radar—in most circles, completely. These very questions are central to our human condition, to our way of living, to our relationships and how we, all of us, feel and function. How can they be *missing in action* in a mental health practice, especially if such questions are essential elements in the very foundations of mental health?

The following questions arise with urgency. *What are we, mental health professionals, doing? And why? What are we thinking? And why? What are the underlying presuppositions guiding our practices? And why? And what are the consequences of this, leading to the state of affairs just described, when those suffering are not getting helped sufficiently—or worse?* Do we need to re-think our approach to mental health and the foundations on which it is built? Do we need to re-build from the ground up?

CHAPTER 2

Current practices and corrupt science

Once you label me you negate me.
Søren Kierkegaard

A phenomenon within the professional mental health field is the proliferation of new therapies on a regular basis. Many take an aspect of psychotherapy or psychoanalysis, cognitive or behavioural psychology, psychiatry, or some combination, and turn it into a new thing. "Science" is routinely invoked as the gold standard of practice. Sometimes new key terms (jargon) are employed. There is a great deal of old wine being poured into new bottles. While some wines improve with air to breathe once opened, even the best wine will go off with too much. The result is a crowded, messy, and fragmented field of mental health practices that is confusing to both patients and professionals. How is anyone ever to figure out what is best for them?

Some practitioners think they will enhance their effectiveness if they learn an ever-growing repertoire of techniques and therapeutic approaches. There are hundreds. Which one to choose?

The results of research into which is the best therapeutic modality vary considerably, and sometimes contradictory results cancel each other out. There is little consistency, and often vested interests and agendas colour the canvas or distort its interpretation. Some research studies are done well and provide valuable information, but the results of some studies are understated, exaggerated, or wholly misrepresented. Then, in practice, patients turn up saying they have different diagnoses from different mental health professionals and treatment results are inconsistent. These differences exist not only between psychiatrists and psychologists but also between one psychiatrist and another, and between one psychologist and another.

Current practices compete to be top dog in the field of mental health. Professionals easily become ideologically invested in the medical model and rationalise its validity especially through the appropriation of scientific methodologies. Psychology and psychiatry are not exact sciences, although they are promoted as such. What is needed is not a more rigorous research methodology to produce a greater volume of "scientific" peer-reviewed studies but rather a more philosophical inquiry into the very presupposition that diagnosis and treatment in mental health should be based on medical science. A key question here is: *What does it mean to be a person?*

Current practices

The major current mainstream practices are psychology and psychiatry. Psychology is defined as the study of behaviour although etymologically the word suggests it is more the study (Gk: *logos*) of the soul or mind (Gk: *psyche*). The term "psychology" is a broad umbrella that encompasses many mental health practices including psychotherapy, psychoanalysis, psychiatry, counselling, mental health nursing, and so on. These days the term "psychology" is used in a narrower sense, almost exclusively to refer to *academic* psychology, where researchers have pioneered methods based on cognitive and behavioural psychology that are subsumed under the label cognitive behavioural therapy or CBT.

Psychiatry is etymologically the *healing* of the soul (Gk: *iatros*—healer, physician). It involves a range of "healing" practices, including medication, electro-convulsive therapy, psychosurgery, hospitalisation, or some combination. Psychotherapy and psychology are part of psychiatry training, and some psychiatrists are more drawn to talk therapy than to churning fifteen-minute consultations to adjust medications. Listening to patients takes time and private psychiatrists charge by the part-hour. There is an inherent conflict of interest when you can make so much more money by not listening! The situation has been made more confusing by changes that allow some psychologists to prescribe medications. I find it astonishing how many of my patients take antidepressants, anxiolytics, anti-psychotics, and mood stabilisers, the major groups of psychiatric medications. No wonder the pharmaceutical industry is booming, surely another indicator of the epidemic crisis in mental health. Medication can be life-saving, yet sometimes I wonder if prescribers benefit more from medicating the suffering of others than patients do. Another short cut?

Despite some broad differences, psychology and psychiatry share a fundamental affinity; both aspire to the status of a science. "Evidence" is now such a buzz word that the prevailing view is that like medical science, psychological practices *should be* evidence-based. After all, evidence shows what works and what doesn't, evidence defines effectiveness and best practice and limits the potential consequences of practice. There is nothing fundamentally wrong with basing therapy practice upon evidence if the evidence has been determined honestly, free from bias, prejudice, and vested interest. It also doesn't work if evidence has been derived from an overly reductive approach. On this point, Nancy McWilliams says that we cannot limit our assessment of improvements to the "evidence" based on symptom reduction alone, but by changes in general life satisfaction, attachment security, authenticity, emotion tolerance and regulation, resilience, capacity to reflect on the self, capacity to "mentalize" others, flexibility of response to stress, vitality, acceptance of what cannot be changed, and other aspects of overall psychological health (e.g., Kanfer & Goldstein, 1991; Luborsky, 1984; Strupp & Hadley, 1977). (2017, p. 286)

The issue is not that psychotherapy shouldn't be *based on* research, rather this is different from psychotherapy being *like* research.

The current pressures on therapists to define a patient's suffering using a single categorical label, to take objective measures, to manualize what one does, to work in the shortest framework possible, and to judge improvement by symptomatic change constitute the misapplication of a research paradigm to a clinical one, a category mistake. (2017, p. 286, original emphasis)

The question of evidence takes us back to the issue: *What does it mean to be a person?* In physical medicine, there is no issue about separating out and isolating physicality from any other aspect of being a person. We accept this. We take it for granted. This is bio-medicine in all its glorious limitations. And it works—as far as it goes. It works in so far as your physical body needs investigating, treating, and repairing. I am grateful to physical medicine for multiple repairs, surgical interventions, and almost certainly saving my life. Sometimes, a person needs *only* something physical. In psychotherapy, however, we rarely see patients with one discrete disorder and not comorbid with anything else. In contrast with physical medicine, the person of the therapy patient is usually highly complex and their complexity has everything to do with the nature of their mental condition and emotional suffering. For this reason, if I felt mentally unwell, my doctor would not be my first port of call.

I need to qualify this. Doctors do help patients with mental unwellness—of course. Some offer counselling though the quality varies greatly. All offer medication, some more judiciously than others. Medication for mental unwellness is a contentious subject. Even so, if I have a patient that is suicidally depressed and "high risk" then I do engage their general medical practitioner or a psychiatrist or hospital. There are moments where such interventions are indispensable and lifesaving. (It is also a good time to have psychotherapy, if possible.)

That said, it is highly questionable that evidence for psychiatry and psychology should be used in the same manner as physical medicine. It is bad enough that physical medicine itself strips away so much of what it means to be a *person* to treat the body as a thing-in-itself—despite the many benefits of this, as I've said. To do the same with mental disorders is a disaster and confuses the forms and processes of mental disorders with physical disorders. Even speaking about mental and physical disorders as two separate "things" is problematic. Mental/emotional suffering invariably affects the body and is affected by the body. What it means to be a *person*, amongst so many things, is to be embodied. While medicine has now accepted that the microbiome of the gut is connected to the brain, this is not the same thing as mind–body inter-relatedness. Much has been said and written about the consequences of dividing mind and body, but have we really taken this on board in our understanding of mental health and the practices that treat it?

If we reduce the understanding and treatment of mental suffering to a science, for example, brain biochemistry or the generalities produced by academic psychological research, the *person* consulting a mental health practitioner is lost and the meaning of their individual suffering is missed.[6] If I am right, this (like the boom in the pharmaceutical industry) begins to point to an answer to the question of why mental disorders exist in epidemic proportions when there has never been so much psychology and psychiatry available to treat them.[7]

I do not dismiss neuroscience and psychobiology. There is a great deal being discovered that has informed our discussions and practices of mental health. I find it interesting. Now we know that well-established neuronal pathways in the brain associated with patterns of experience and behaviour that correspond with mental suffering can be changed (thanks to neuroplasticity) by the ongoing positive experiences generated by an effective therapeutic relationship and process. Great! Moreover, neuroscience and psychobiology have contributed to the development of trauma-informed therapy, so important in the contemporary mental health landscape. Few patients consult us, whatever prompts their seeking help at the outset, without some historical, often childhood trauma—to varying degrees. Often, there are essential connections to be made between the past and the present. Trauma-informed therapy has developed a useful language and understanding that has contributed to improving therapy practices. The principles and practices of trauma-informed therapy are fundamental to good, safe, effective psychotherapy practice. All therapy practice should be trauma-informed.[8]

For all the advances of neuroscience, such developments have barely changed the way I work following my psychotherapy training in the 1970s. What has been most interesting is how much of what I was trained in, accumulated clinical wisdom about what works in psychotherapy, is confirmed by modern science. The contemporary language developed around trauma, shame, dissociation, and clinical process informed by neuroscience and psychobiology were already largely there. Read R. D. Laing, whose best work was written in the 1960s. Laing's work is trauma-informed. Indeed, he was highly sensitised to trauma, having grown up with his own. Of course, my own practice has evolved since the 1970s. We must change and adjust

---

[6] Contrary to this view is the interesting work done by Louis Castonguay and his associates; Castonguay & Muran (2015); Castonguay, Youn, Xiao, Muran, & Barber (2015); Castonguay, Constantino, & Beutler (2019).

[7] In addition, many psychiatrists are now refusing to accept high-risk patients because of the risk to themselves of medico-legal consequences. One psychiatrist told me he felt "hunted" by his patients looking for a possible financial benefit via litigation. This is the case locally; I don't know if it applies elsewhere or to what extent.

[8] See the important publication by Kezelman and Stavropoulos (2012) which can be downloaded for free at https://www.blueknot.org.au/

with the culture—or we fall out of step. While cultural values have everything to do with what is regarded as normative in mental health, we also need to think critically and assess whether cultural trends are themselves healthy or bring consequences. This is also where critical thinking is indispensable.

Keeping in step with culture is a double-edged sword. It has value but sometimes we *need* to fall out of step. Psychoanalysis, for example, has always identified as a subversive practice from its earliest Freudian origins. Some repressive, self-limiting, conventional, and conformist elements in culture need to be subverted and overcome in the interest of developing a strong sense of self, authenticity, agency, creativity, and meaningful pursuits. Psychology and psychiatry have been mainly concerned with assisting patients to adapt to cultural norms, which may or may not be helpful. Following this path can lead to the pathologising of human suffering when people do not fit in, which creates a compound issue: you are not only bad and wrong for not complying with societal norms but now you are mentally ill as well. Being different is not a disease—a point especially important in an era of dawning realisation of how many people are neuro-atypical.

Being different is not a disease.

There are now any number of ways of organising different kinds of mental suffering. The dominant manual in psychiatry is *The Diagnostic and Statistical Manual of the American Psychiatric Association* (DSM) which has been a major influence on what is regarded as normal, or abnormal, in mental health. The DSM is a classificatory system. In one way of looking at it, it merely organises patterns of so-called mental disorders into syndromes for the purposes of diagnosis. However, the language of the DSM also tells another story. Words like *diagnosis* imply a medical condition, and medical means physical. The first paragraph of the Preface to the current edition includes the following statement:

> Since a complete description of the underlying pathological processes is not possible for most mental disorders, it is important to emphasize that the current diagnostic criteria are the best available description of how mental disorders are expressed and can be recognized by trained clinicians. (DSM-5, 2013, p. xli)

"Underlying pathological processes" is exactly the sort of language revealing the thinking behind DSM classifications. Pathology is from the Greek, "science of diseases". Pathological processes happen in the body, but it is not possible, the DSM admits, to apply this to most mental disorders—because they are different. Yet, we still endeavour to diagnose and treat mental disorders as if they were the same as those pathological processes in the body. They are not the same.

This is the very presumptive correlation that becomes confused with causation that requires greater critical scrutiny. The net effect is one where patients become *pathologised* for all manner of affective, cognitive, and behavioural issues depending upon an individual practitioner's view of normal or abnormal psychology. I have been supervising a group of consultant psychiatrists that mainly practice psychotherapy and once when I walked in the room to begin a session, I heard them refer to psychiatry's bible as "the Dumb Stupid Manual" (DSM). Snide jokes aside, are mental disorders medical conditions?

Psychology proceeds along similar lines of diagnosis and treatment and regards the categorisation of mental disorders in the DSM as gospel, unquestioned facts. Why is it so hard for us to think? Mental health practitioners need to think critically as opposed to reducing the most complex issues of mental emotional distress and disorder to a tidy box of generalised descriptions, to which they can give labels, that in turn indicate treatments, and expect the job is done. Most treatments in psychiatry amount to drug treatments; in psychology, there are applied psychological techniques, groups, and psychoeducation, among other strategies.

Are the DSM-based diagnoses applied today consistent over time, as is often the case for physical conditions known through evidence-based research? The point is for people to change, not remain one "thing", and indeed people do change often independently of us, their mental health practitioners. If you are a clinician, surely you have noticed that your patient is very different this week from last week. Last week, you were convinced your patient had borderline personality disorder (that overused and maligned label). This week, just a little narcissistic. Oh, but that laughter, maybe manic? Is speaking that fast normal? I wonder if bi-polar? Would that be bi-polar I or II? What if my patient had a moment of happiness? Is that okay?

Give them a survey, the score will settle it. Do scores give an accurate picture of a person's experience? To answer this question, I gave myself the widely used *Depression, Anxiety and Stress* (DASS-21) questionnaire. I do realise that questionnaires are a kind of shorthand, or preliminary indicator—but indicator of what? Apparently, I am on the cusp of mild to no depression, moderately anxious, and mildly stressed. However, if you simply asked me, I would say that I am not depressed, anxious, or stressed at all. I feel good today, unlike some days.

Let's look at a further example in greater detail—the *Generalised Anxiety Disorder* (GAD-7) scale. I acknowledge the use of such scales is not to draw a conclusion but nevertheless I am questioning the value of a short cut at all. Is it even a short cut if it leads you astray? Over the last two weeks, how often have you been bothered by the following problems?

1) Feeling nervous, anxious, or on edge
2) Not being able to stop or control worrying
3) Worrying too much about different things
4) Trouble relaxing
5) Being so restless that it's hard to sit still
6) Becoming easily annoyed or irritable
7) Feeling afraid as if something awful might happen.

In four columns the scale is

a) Not at all sure
b) Several days
c) Over half the days
d) Nearly every day.

Then you count the days and arrive at a number. Five, ten, and fifteen are cut-off points for mild, moderate, or severe anxiety. When ten or greater, further investigation is needed.

To me, if you did this scale on one day and then consulted a different mental health professional a fortnight later, you may well have different answers. If you did this scale in the morning and consulted the same mental health professional in the afternoon or evening, you might get a different score. If you consulted a different mental health professional on the same day and did the questions again, you might get a different score because you feel differently with the second person than with the first. Maybe the first reminds you of your father, with whom you had a poor relationship, and the second reminds you of your mother, with whom you had a good relationship. Maybe you liked the first but didn't like the second. Maybe you felt more anxious with the second but felt soothed by the first. Maybe you disliked both but always feel worse in the mornings. And so on. Is it not surprising that people turn up with different scores, depending on a long list of variables?

Further, if you ask me how many days in the last fortnight I had trouble relaxing, worried too much, or became annoyed or irritable—I would have no idea. What's too much? I don't count days of worry. Surely, my annoyance depends on what is happening. I can get annoyed at the traffic light turning red, yet sometimes nothing annoys me. Maybe I don't have a generalised anxiety disorder but sometimes life seems like a generalised anxiety disorder!

Psychology practice follows the same structure of diagnosis and treatment as psychiatry. Training in psychology typically proceeds via statistics and research methodologies. Indeed, in Australia, countless psychology undergraduates leave university disillusioned because they had thought they were learning a clinical discipline. They wanted to become a psychologist to help people and leave as statisticians and researchers with little understanding of people.

Despite having a PhD in Psychology, focused on the interface between psychosomatics and psychoanalysis, I was refused registration as a psychologist when I came to Australia in 1990 because I hadn't studied statistics, psychometric testing, and quantitative research methodology at undergraduate level. Instead, I had studied European Continental Philosophy, Existentialism, and Phenomenology—all of which have proved invaluable in my psychotherapy practice. The Psychologists Board had been stopping therapists and counsellors from practising if they hadn't followed the mainstream psychology pathway and then registered as a psychologist and so tried to stop me. I litigated to advocate for my rights and those of others unfairly excluded and sometimes persecuted, and long story short the Board withdrew from the case. They must have been told by their lawyers they had been indulging in restrictive practices following a prejudicial interpretation of the relevant act. This marked the beginning of a legitimate psychotherapy profession in Western Australia (circa 1993). I wound up becoming the Founding President of the Psychotherapists and Counsellors Association of Western Australia.

This is far from an isolated example of professionals acting restrictively and attempting to monopolise the professional field in the service of their own agendas. It has nothing to do with science or the kind of evidence one can derive from a limited study of a small sample of people whose scores on various instruments are handled statistically. In contrast, some excellent work has been done by such notable figures as Jonathan Shedler in the USA, and Farhad Dalal and Joanna Moncrieff in England. In what follows, I refer to their work to show examples of corruption in the politics, science, and research methods that have contributed to the proliferation of ineffectual approaches to mental health.

Corrupt science

Behaviour therapy, having made its reputation treating phobias, later joined forces with the emerging field of cognitive psychology. While not the most compatible bedfellows, they had a common agenda: to counter the domination of psychoanalytic therapies most prevalent in the 1960s. Fast forward to the contemporary scene of a mental health epidemic, CBT has positioned itself out of all proportion as the gold standard treatment for all manner of mental disorders. They have been successful in this spin of mythology but not without a litany of problems, and failings, in its wake. Jonathan Shedler (2017) says if you actually read the original sources of research, you discover a vast difference between what research shows and what we are told it shows. CBT has been oversold; the evidence for its efficacy has been wildly misrepresented.

In one study, that compared a type of CBT with psychodynamic psychotherapy for post-traumatic stress disorder (PTSD) following simple trauma in adolescents, the conclusion drawn by investigators and widely published (originally in a top-tier research journal) was that CBT was superior to psychodynamic psychotherapy in decreasing symptoms of depression, enhancing functioning, and in leading to overall improvement. If you only read the title, the abstract, and the conclusion—or simply a report of this study—you would come away with this belief (Shedler, 2017).

So, who were these psychodynamic psychotherapists who participated in this "gold standard" randomly controlled trial? It turns out they were graduate students and given two days of training—by another graduate student. Amazingly, the psychodynamic psychotherapists were forbidden to discuss the trauma that brought the patient for therapy in the first place. They were instructed to change the subject. Remember: this is a trial comparing the efficacy of treatment for post-traumatic stress disorder following one instance of trauma—but "Do not discuss the trauma".

In the registered training organisation that I ran for 18 years, The Churchill Clinic, where we conferred nationally accredited post-graduate degrees, the average time to qualify as a psychodynamic psychotherapist was seven years, following intensive study, personal therapy, extensive clinical supervision, seminars, workshops, and lectures all delivered by senior clinicians, and sometimes leading international figures who visited. Looking more closely at the evidence base of CBT, the only conclusion I can draw is that it is a lie that serves as fuel for a massive, and highly effective marketing campaign (Shedler, 2017).

Shedler says you might think he is cherry-picking the odd example of questionable research and reporting to suit his own purposes. However, a comprehensive review of psychotherapy from the *Clinical Psychology Review* looked at all the randomised-control studies available for anxiety and depression with a control group. They looked at 2,500 abstracts and then narrowed that down to 149 relevant studies that compared an evidence-based treatment with another established treatment. They found only fourteen of those actually compared an evidence-based treatment to something approaching a legitimate control group.

Their conclusion was that most of the treatments being compared with CBT involved no psychotherapy whatsoever. Where psychotherapy had been included, the therapists were prevented from delivering therapy in the manner they normally would. Shedler repeats again: the control groups were a sham. The conclusion of this study was: there is insufficient evidence to suggest that transporting an evidence-based therapy to routine care that already involves psychotherapy will improve the quality of services (Shedler, 2017).

> "Evidence-based therapies have *not* shown 'superiority' to any other legitimate psychotherapy, and that is a scientific fact."
>
> (Jonathan Shedler, 2017)

That is also the conclusion of the American Psychological Association: evidence-based therapies have not shown any greater benefit than any other form of psychotherapy (Shedler, 2017).

In a book that has received widespread acclaim, and deservedly so, the unfortunately titled *CBT: The Cognitive Behavioural Tsunami* and subtitled *Managerialism, Politics and the Corruptions of Science* (2018) Farhad Dalal lays bare the underlying distortions and manipulations of research yielding the "evidence" of mainstream psychology. He asserts that the definition of "evidence" as used in psychological research is a "hyper-rationalist reality" and by becoming the ruling definition, it dismisses other types of evidence. For example, if you ask me "*On a scale of one to ten how depressed do you feel?*" and I answer "*I feel a six*", then that number counts as objective data and therefore qualifies as evidence. If I add "*As soon as I answered I noticed I felt quite a lot better*", that doesn't count as "evidence" because it is merely anecdotal and hence, subjective. There is no number: "… *in order for something to count, it has to be countable*" (Dalal, 2018, p. 4).

CBT has evolved over its history via a series of waves. The first wave (in the 1920s) was behaviourism, the second wave (1960s) added on cognition and largely focused on changing what was regarded as errors in your thinking. You might well ask who decides what is an error and what is not? Or who decides what I should think or not think? Who decides who decides? The third wave has gone Buddhist and emphasises accepting what goes on inside. I understand a more recent wave has some CBT psychologists interested in affect. The language has changed and words like mindfulness, attachment, compassion, and acceptance are in vogue.

I am a fan of all these words but to imply that psychology has invented them is dishonest and misleading. For me, turning these concepts into techniques and training people to regard therapy as an application of them is a bastardisation of the very traditions from which they are derived. The words lose their meanings in the bargain. Dalal puts it thus:

> In effect, the philosophy and practice of Mindfulness has been colonised by the device of giving it the gloss of "Science". Knowledge and expertise no longer reside with monks and mendicants who have put in lifetimes of practice to achieve something akin to the state of Mindfulness. Now all one has to do is to take a twelve-week course to achieve the same ends.
>
> In proceeding this way, not only have these practices been instrumentalized, but worse the end to which they have been instrumentalized is a perversion of the very philosophies that generated them. In Eastern philosophies, the purpose of meditative practices is to help the meditator to work towards the state of Nirvana, which requires the dissolution of the Self. In CBT practice, Mindfulness and the like are being used in the service of reinforcing the Self. But worse is to follow. In the very same breath as mentioning the Buddha, Layard, and Clark celebrate the fact that, "The Resilience Programme" [which utilizes mindfulness] is now being used for every soldier in the US Army, with the aim of reducing the incidence of post-traumatic stress disorder after traumatic experiences on the battlefield' (Layard and Clark, 2014, p. 230).
>
> In other words, the Buddhist practice of mindfulness is being used to turn human beings into more efficient, more resilient, killing machines. (2018, p. 38)

When psychologists accept the premises and definitions of DSM, they ignore or trivialise the personal reasons for or social causes of mental disorder. Context is irrelevant; all that matters is what keeps a condition going and how to cure it.

From the perspective of many academic psychologists, if someone keeps lighting unwanted fires, knowledge of what motivates them doesn't help put out the fires. For psychotherapists, if someone keeps lighting unwanted fires, we need to understand their reasons for doing so and the context in which this occurs to consider how to help them stop themselves from lighting fires. Psychotherapy is focused upon the meaning of experience and behaviour. Efforts by many psychologists and psychiatrists to get rid of meaning as a consideration in treatment have had devastating consequences on real people. Talk about chalk and cheese; it is hard to believe these professions—psychotherapy, psychology, psychiatry—are working in the same realm of mental health, disorder, and the relief of suffering. They could hardly be more different.

I don't think exploring the meaning of an experience or a behaviour involving the lighting of fires needs to preclude us from trying to help put them out. If I can help a patient feel less depressed or anxious before I have any idea as to why they feel that way or what it means, I am all for it. In fact, I'm for anything that works within reason. Yet, clinical experience shows time and again that whether a psychotherapist or a psychologist or anyone else helps a person feel less depressed or anxious (or whatever) on any given occasion, if that person has a tendency towards depression or anxiety (or whatever) it is likely they will return there. It is a matter of time. Such patterns require an investigation of the origins and reasons for it, and context is essential for a meaningful understanding. Sometimes that is enough to engender a lasting improvement and sometimes it isn't. Explaining and understanding do not necessarily change patterns. This is why therapy outcomes can require a long-term process of growth and development through an ongoing professional relationship and is rarely achieved by short-term techniques and methods, whatever alphabet soup of acronyms is served: ACT, CBT, CFT, DBT, EFT, EMDR, FAP, MCT, and so on.

As noted, the base stock of the alphabet soup of psychology is the DSM which has been revised many times. DSM-5 states that "past science was not mature enough to yield fully validated diagnoses—that is, to provide consistent, strong, and objective validators of individual DSM disorders" (2013, p. 5). This implies present science is mature enough. With some humility, the Introduction to DSM-5 goes on to admit:

> the boundaries between many disorder "categories" are more fluid over the life course than DSM-IV recognized, and many symptoms assigned to a single disorder may occur, at varying levels of severity, in many other disorders. (2013, p. 5)

And later:

> we have come to recognize that the boundaries between disorders are more porous than originally perceived. (2013, p. 6)

This is not surprising given that DSM-I (1952) listed 106 disorders, DSM-II (1968) listed 182 disorders, DSM-III (1980) listed 265 disorders, DSM-IV (1994) listed 297 disorders, and then the manual was revised in DSM-IV-TR (2000) and now DSM-5 (2013). Due to complaints about the ever-growing number of mental disorders, no increase occurred in DSM-5. However, closer inspection reveals this was achieved by making several disorders subsets of other disorders and therefore the overall number has not increased. We can do many things to manipulate numbers to create a desired impression. I wonder how many mental disorders will "exist" in 2050?

"Fully validated diagnoses" is an interesting expression. Spitzer (the principal author of DSM-III, and its revolutionary turn away from any psychodynamic influence of the previous editions to a more biologically based view) claimed that "drafts of the DSM were tested in field trials involving over 12,000 patients and 550 clinicians in 212 different facilities" (1980, p. 5). According to Dalal "there is no evidence for this momentous claim" (2018, p. 53). Sometimes the evidence base lacks any trace of evidence at all.

The historical background to this "revolutionary turning" was that psychiatrists were unhappy that non-medical "competitors" offering psychodynamically based therapies at lower fees motivated the psychiatric profession to adopt the position that its diagnoses were of more consistent, medically based illnesses, and therefore more efficacious. At the same time, governments and insurance providers were unhappy that the non-medical, psychodynamic approaches were not uniform in their classification of disorders and so indulged in longer-term, theoretically unnecessary therapies, thereby creating excessive expenditure (Kawa & Giordano, 2012). This also opened the door for the advent of psychometric testing, quantitative assessments, rating scales, and the various checklists for anxiety and depression. When you look more closely at the underlying reasons for mental health structures as we find them today, the drivers are largely cultural; they are based on commercial interests and professional competition. Science has been bent to fit cultural and professional agendas.

As an example, one of the great historical confusions around fully validated disorders relates to homosexuality. It was long thought of as an illness in psychology, psychiatry, and psychoanalysis and so was included in DSM-II under the heading "Sexual Deviation Disorder". Rising cultural discontent put sufficient pressure on this classification so that in DSM-III homosexuality was identified as an "Ego-Dystonic Disorder". This is a long way from a sexual deviation; rather, feeling unhappy being gay is the problem, not the gayness itself. Nevertheless, homosexuality remained tarred with the brush of pathology (notice the medicalisation here of sexual orientation). When DSM-III was revised, the R edition removed homosexuality entirely. This is primarily a response to the cultural values and ideologies of the day. I think culture has everything to do with what we regard as a disorder or not—let's be honest about it—and not pretend such values are *fully* validated by scientific research.

Dalal points out that once homosexuality had been removed from the DSM, immigration laws had to be changed (in the United States) from those that excluded the naturalisation of gay people on the grounds that it was a diagnosable condition *according to the DSM*. Such is the political power of this document. He goes on to discuss PTSD, which didn't exist until the 1960s and 1970s.[9]

---

[9] In a private communication, Nancy McWilliams pointed out that, initially, we didn't have PTSD by this name but there were numerous descriptors such as "war neuroses", "shell shock", and "battle fatigue" from past wars. "The real revolution was Judith Herman's argument that sexual abuse of children was just as psychologically devastating as the experiences of war and disaster that has come to be called PTSD in the 1960s."

For me, this descriptor is too restrictive in its definition as a diagnostic category. To me, trauma brings a multitude of consequences that often last a long time. This view is real-world, practice-based, and self-evident. There is a vast range of issues—comorbidities if you like—and a broad range of variation in how so-called PTSD unfolds over a long time frame, maybe a lifetime.

To qualify for benefits, soldiers returning from the Vietnam War needed a psychiatric disorder to be diagnosed. Dalal says that Spitzer initially resisted its inclusion in the DSM because it violated "basic guidelines about theory and research that had been established for DSM-III" (2018, p. 56). The new manual set out to omit causes from their description of disorders and obviously PTSD is inherently linked with trauma as its cause.

> When PTSD was first introduced into the DSM-III, those who were deemed subject to this "mental disorder" were traumatized soldiers. In other words, those who were traumatised primarily through being the *perpetrators* of violence. But in DSM-IV, PTSD shape-shifted and its focus became centred entirely on the victims of violence (accidents, domestic and sexual abuse and so forth). While this shift is not unreasonable in itself, it did not come about because of scientific research, but rather through the advocacy of various pressure groups.
>
> In sum, the story of PTSD not only shows up the vacuity of the claim that its contents of the DSM are scientific but also reveals that the DSM is the gate through which all must pass before they will be given a hearing by the legislature and the authorities generally. (Dalal, 2018, p. 57)

I am not the only professional who has issues with the concept of PTSD. Judith Herman, professor of psychiatry at Harvard University in her book *Trauma and Recovery* (1992, p. 121) proposed a new syndrome of C-PTSD referring to complex trauma, since PTSD alone typically refers to simple or singular trauma. She rightly argues people that have suffered extreme and repetitious trauma tend to suffer a broad range of manifest consequences including those affecting:

- Affect (especially shame, guilt, and self-blame)
- Consciousness including memory, hyper-vigilance, dissociation
- Self-perception
- Perception of others especially the perpetrator
- Relationships
- Systems of meaning
- Bodily functioning and experiencing, hyper- or hypo-arousal
- Mood, cognitive functioning
- Sleep disorders including nightmares
- Sexuality.[10]

---

[10] I have expanded the list she provides.

There is a disjunction between simple trauma that may inform a diagnosis of PTSD, and complex and prolonged trauma and the multiple issues for treatment that takes the full scope of what complex trauma means into account.

* * *

Psychiatry, as noted above, sets out to follow general medicine. In this regard, Joanna Moncrieff, a British psychiatrist, senior lecturer at University College, London, and leading figure in the Critical Psychiatry movement, makes a distinction between a disease-centred model of drug action and a drug-centred model in her book *The Bitterest Pills: The Troubling Story of Antipsychotic Drugs* (2013). The disease-centred model is a particular way of understanding the action of psychiatric drugs, but not the only way and not necessarily the best. Indeed, to her, it is not even a correct way.

> The disease-centred model of drug action is based on the idea that drugs work by acting on the aberrant biological processes, be it chemical imbalances or other abnormalities, which are assumed to produce the symptoms of a particular disorder. According to this view, drugs make the body more "normal" by helping to reverse an underlying disease or dysfunction. This action on the disease process is the drug's "therapeutic" action and all its other actions are designated as "side effects" and considered to be of secondary importance.
>
> The disease-centred model is borrowed from general medicine, where most modern drugs act on the physiological pathways that produce the symptoms of a disease. (Moncrieff, 2013, pp. 8–9)

Moreover:

> The disease-centred model of drug action has become the dominant way of theorizing what drugs do when they are taken by someone with a mental health problem. It is so influential that people are not aware that there are other ways of conceptualising how drugs affect people with mental disorders, or whether the disease-centred model is supported by scientific evidence. But the idea that psychiatric drugs work by targeting underlying biological processes that are specific to certain sorts of mental health problems or symptoms is central to the way that psychiatric treatment is administered and presented, and to the way that research on drug treatment is designed, conducted, and interpreted. (2013, p. 9)

And referring to the latest edition of a principal American textbook of psychiatry, she observes that it stresses mental disorders are true medical conditions that can benefit from drug therapy in the same way that diabetes, asthma and hypothyroidism, and other chronic disorders are responsive to medication. (2013, p. 9)

She says chemical imbalances are *assumed* to produce the symptoms of a disorder. That doesn't sound like medical *science*.

In contrast to the disease-centred model, the drug-centred model understands drugs as drugs, first and foremost. In other words, drugs affect the body whatever condition the body is in, whatever symptoms are being experienced, and whatever one's mental state. Because psychiatric drugs are psychoactive, they affect how the brain functions and therefore these drugs are designed to change mental experience and functioning. Changes in behaviour follow.

You might well be wondering: what is the difference between legal medicines inducing altered states and recreational drugs like LSD, MDMA, psylocibin (magic mushrooms), cocaine, ketamine, cannabis, methamphetamine, heroin, or everyday drugs like nicotine, caffeine, and alcohol? All are affecting, if not intoxicating, to a greater or lesser degree. Substances are taken voluntarily to make you feel better than your "natural" state. Some, like cannabis, are legalised increasingly. And others, like psylocibin and MDMA, are being researched because of therapeutic benefits and may be legalised for medical use in the future—especially for PTSD. Moncrieff is arguing that the aim of psychoactive psychiatric medications is largely to induce an altered state and not treat an underlying disease process, as is usually claimed. The aim is to make you feel different, and ideally *better*. She has spent much of her career researching psychiatric medications. In *The Myth of the Antidepressant: An Historical Analysis* (2011) one of her conclusions is expressed as:

> Most research on the history of psychiatry has accepted the portrayal of modern psychiatric drugs as specific of disease-centred agents. Hence drugs are often credited with revolutionizing psychiatry by bringing it in line with medical science and breaking the influence of psychoanalysis and social psychiatry (Shorter, 1997).
>
> However, there is little evidence to support the assumption that psychiatric drugs act in a specific, disease-centred manner (Moncrieff & Cohen, 2005, 2006). In the case of antidepressants, recent meta-analyses suggest that their advantage over a placebo is small, and possibly clinically meaningless (Kirsch et al., 2002; Kirsch, this volume; NICE, 2004), and it has never been demonstrated that they have consistently superior effects to other drugs with psychoactive properties. Contrary to popular belief, it has *not* been demonstrated that depression is associated with an abnormality or imbalance of serotonin, or *any other* brain chemical, or that drugs act by reversing such a problem (Moncrieff & Cohen, 2006). (Moncrieff, 2011, pp. 176–177, original emphasis)

This is worth repeating:

> "It has *not* been demonstrated that depression is associated with an abnormality or imbalance of serotonin, or *any other* brain chemical, or that drugs act by reversing such a problem."

Why are so many doctors and mental health professionals propagating this mythology, singing Big Pharma's song?

Even the term "antidepressant" seems to have been invented with little evidence to support the myth that there is a drug that can target a specific chemical imbalance that accounts for the supposed medical condition of depression. Depression is a real condition of mental ill-health. Indeed, depression is one of the worst states of mind there is, characterised by low mood, inertia, dysphoria, and, at worst, suicidality. At its worst, there is psycho-motor retardation, a very physical condition, as well as cognitive impairment, a mental condition. There are probably chemical imbalances or irregularities in the brain, and elsewhere in the body, that correspond with depressed states of mind. *But correlation is not causation.*

So many interests and agendas are served:

- the psychiatry profession seeking to be regarded as prestigious medical professionals
- the pharmaceutical industry wanting to generate an enormous market for its products[11]
- government pursuing simple solutions to complex social problems.

Mental health professionals are disadvantaged to pursue the underlying personal, social, familial, and historic reasons that underlie depression—and other mental health conditions—independently of any biological correlates that may or may not exist. I am not against medication for such conditions. Medications help people sometimes, to some degree. I am against the kind of misinformation that hoodwinks ordinary people into believing they have a medical condition characterised by a chemical imbalance effectively treated by a medication that corrects it. Common acceptance of a lie does not make it true. All of us have a big mountain to climb if we are to overcome the post-truth tendencies of our shared culture and work towards honesty and integrity as the core of our professional lives.

Moncrieff, in discussing the "evidence" behind the concept of the drug imipramine, the first "antidepressant medication", says:

---

[11] Dalal says the pharmaceutical industry spends twice as much money on marketing as on research (2018, p. 92) and sponsors ninety per cent of the published clinical trials which, in turn, support the declared efficacy of its own products (2018, p. 60)!

there was, and remains, no evidence to suggest that imipramine and other antidepressant drugs act in a disease-centred fashion on the biological basis of depressant symptoms.

This challenges the conventional view of the recent history of psychiatry, which suggests that modern day drugs helped to transform psychiatry into a genuine scientific activity. This view is premised on the idea that modern drugs are disease- or symptom-specific treatments; that they work by reversing some or all of an underlying physical pathology. It is the idea of the *specificity of action* that makes drug treatment *appear* to be a therapeutic, medical enterprise. If, in contrast, modern psychiatric treatments are not specific, if they act merely by inducing psychoactive effects that suppress or contain psychiatric distress and problematic behaviours, then psychiatry has not moved far from its historical roots as a superficially, or metaphorically medicalized form of social control. (2011, pp. 187–188, original emphasis)

And further along:

Over the last 20 years, many millions of people around the world have been persuaded that their difficulties arise from a brain disorder that can be called "depression" and corrected by drug treatment. The ideas of "depression" and "antidepressants" have been marketed, as "diseases", to a general audience as never before. Few people are aware that these concepts have their origins, not in robust scientific research, but rather in the interests of a psychiatric profession desperate to cement its professional position, and in the marketing tactics of the pharmaceutical industry. Antidepressants have transformed a myriad of social and personal problems into a source of corporate profit and professional prestige. (2011, p. 188)

Dalal picks up the theme of research into antidepressants in his discussion of the corruptions of science. He claims that deceitful and self-serving practices have become the norm of what passes for scientific psychological research. A group of researchers tracked all registered clinical trials for all the antidepressants launched between 1987 and 2004:

38 of the trials concluded that the treatment being tested worked, and 36 found that the treatment did not. 37 of the 38 trials with positive results were published, whilst only 3 out the 36 negative trials were. Of the remaining 33 trials with negative outcomes, 22 never saw the light of day again, and quite astonishingly, the remaining 11 were written up as if the drug were a success. Consequently, when doctors looked to the published "research" to help make an informed decision, they found 48 trials had apparently demonstrated the efficacy of anti-depressants, set against 3 that did not. The published evidence make it appear that the efficacy of anti-depressants was uncontroversial. (2018, p. 154)

Shedler echoes this sentiment in his comments about "publication bias", saying that effect sizes for CBT (the claimed benefits for depression) were exaggerated or inflated by seventy-five per cent, which means that the *actual* benefit is about one quarter of what the literature would suggest (2017).

Therein lies corruption, a misuse of "science" in the service of vested interests. Dalal goes on to say that the Food and Drug Administration (FDA) in the United States throws out the negative results of trials. All they require are two positive trials to approve public use. The standard is so low that it is not hard to achieve a positive result for just about anything if a corporation wants to make a case for it. In discussing the numerous problems besetting research, he concludes:

> This in turn allows all sorts of mischief and mistruth to pass itself off as empirical evidence-based scientific knowledge. (2018, p. 156)

When you hear about the evidence base ensuring that a certain practice is "the gold standard" underpinned by science, listen with a sceptical ear. Catchy slogans and misleading advertising have infiltrated mental health professions. Unfortunately, it is worse than that because to say *correlation is not causation* is to give credence to the existence of correlation; the assumption of correlation takes it for granted. Far too often, correlation has been proven by research only to be comprehensively disproven later by further and more extensive research. It is said that science self-corrects, but in practice, this does not consider the very human psychology of researchers. Specifically, personal and corporate agendas trump the principle of objectivity and impartiality. (This is why analytic/psychodynamic psychotherapy and psychoanalysis focus on desire as the underlying force of motivation.)

I found in the science archives of *The Atlantic* an amazing article by Ed Yong titled "A Waste of 1,000 Research Papers—Decades of Early Research on the Genetics of Depression were Built on Non-Existent Foundations. How Did That Happen?" (2019). In 1996, a certain gene called SLC6A4 was found to be more common in 454 people with mood disorders than 570 that did not. This gene is responsible for generating serotonin and transmitting it into brain cells. One thousand research papers later and a further seventeen genes were linked to depression, with SLC6A4 dominant amongst them. Later, a much larger study with groups of subjects ranging from 62,000 to 443,000 assessed the prevalence of these genes in depressed people. "We didn't find a smidge of evidence", says Matthew Kellerm, who led the project (Yong, 2019). And he added: "This should be a cautionary tale. How on Earth could we have spent 20 years and hundreds of millions of dollars studying pure noise?"

Yong quotes blogger Scott Alexander's reaction:

> What bothers me isn't just that people said [the gene] mattered and it didn't. It's that we built whole imaginary edifices on top of this idea of [it] mattering. (2019)

And referring to the way researchers studied how SLC6A4 affects emotion centres in the brain, how its influence varies in different countries and demographics, and how it interacts with other genes, it's as if they had been describing the life cycle of unicorns, what unicorns eat, all the different subspecies of unicorn, which cuts of unicorn meat are tastiest, and a blow-by-blow account of a wrestling match between unicorns and Bigfoot. (2019)

He says it well. Genetic research has come a long way since then and what has been realised is this: most mental disorders—and most physical diseases for that matter—are affected by huge numbers of genes—thousands—and each gene has a miniscule effect.

Another researcher, initially impressed with the early indications of SLC6A4 research, later realised how insubstantial the evidence was for it to be regarded as having any influence on depression at all. With others, Marcus Munafò of the University of Bristol conducted a much larger study in 2005—but got nothing.

> You would have thought that would have dampened enthusiasm for that particular candidate gene, but not at all. Any evidence that the results might not be reliable was simply not what many people wanted to hear. (Munafò in Yong, 2019)

Wanted to hear—this is what the term "desire" above refers to. This is what people want. He continues:

> We're told that science self-corrects, but what the candidate gene literature demonstrates is that it often self-corrects very slowly, and very wastefully, even when the writing has been on the wall for a very long time. (Munafò in Yong, 2019)

The pace of literature on SLC6A4 and its relation to depression not only didn't slow down after his study disproved any *meaningful* connection at all, but it accelerated. The total number of such papers quadrupled over the next decade. Munafò continues:

> Many fields of science, from psychology to cancer biology, have been dealing with similar problems: Entire lines of research may be based on faulty results. The reasons for this so-called reproducibility crisis are manifold. Sometimes, researchers futz with their data until they get something interesting, or retrofit their questions to match their answers. Other times, they selectively publish positive results while sweeping negative ones under the rug, creating a false impression of building evidence. (Munafò in Yong, 2019)

Also known as post-truth; or, simply, untruth.

In the academic world, researchers are rewarded, indeed celebrated, for making great discoveries and for being productive. It matters more to make a big statement than a correct one. It is better to create a tall building than to check the foundations on which it is built. There is a collective perception that the taller the building, the stronger—but things are not always as they appear. Many geneticists now regard the candidate gene approach as a historical embarrassment that has largely been abandoned. Others have not realised there is even any question as to the validity of this approach and are continuing to research the SLC6A4/candidate gene and its influence upon depression. Who knows what they may discover?

Munafò argues for the sentiment that a culture needs to be developed that motivates and rewards researchers for pursuing true and correct results and he ends with the quote: "Those who don't learn from the past are doomed to repeat it." This quote has been attributed to a 1905 study by the Spanish philosopher George Santayana (possibly anticipated by Edmund Burke, the Anglo-Irish statesman and philosopher, a century-and-a-half earlier). To me, it is ironic that the article ends on such a distinctly Freudian theme.

As noted above, when I first arrived to live and work in Western Australia, I was refused registration as a psychologist. Though I was well-qualified and had had fifteen years in practice by then, I had not gone through the traditional university route of undergraduate studies in statistics, psychometric testing, and quantitative research methodology. I was disdainful of the value of these subjects for clinical practice in psychotherapy (and still am) though they remain academic requirements. However, I thought I should have a better idea of what academic psychology espoused, especially as I had been asked to lead the psychologists' colloquium at some of the local universities. I bought the textbooks used in the undergraduate courses in psychology at the University of Western Australia. One was called *Abnormal Psychology* and the other was a textbook on CBT. I was vaguely comfortable with the first text, though I don't really subscribe to the terms "normal" or "abnormal".

The second textbook was truly disturbing to me. In the whole of the text, the words "love", "sex", "God", and "money" never appeared anywhere. I thought to myself: these are four of the largest categories that bring people to consult me for help. How can there be no reference? What is more, there was also no reference to the major existential questions such as *Why live? What is life for? What are we doing here? What matters? What is the meaning of living?*

We begin to consider such questions when people consult us because they feel empty inside, when they have no motivation or direction, and when a personal sense of purpose eludes them. It is all too easy to diagnose this state of affairs as "depression" but we are travelling in a very personal territory in which statistics, psychometric testing, and bogus evidence have no use. This journey can be depressing but the underlying issue is one of meaning, or, more accurately, the lack of it: *meaninglessness*. It is this issue that I want to explore in the following chapter.

CHAPTER 3

The existential vacuum: meaninglessness and filling the void

There is nothing in the world, I venture to say, that would so effectively help one to survive even the worst conditions as the knowledge that there is a meaning in one's life.
Viktor Frankl

Harold, a therapy patient, came into a session visibly distressed. Over the course of the session, he told me about a friend.

> Bradley was a tall, good looking forty-two-year-old man with his life in good order. He had worked hard as a younger man to qualify as a doctor and then a medical specialist. He belonged to a tight group of friends most of whom he had known for years. He liked outdoor activities, worked out at the gym, swam in the sea, and was careful about his diet. He liked fine dining and was fussy about wine. He would say "I'm a Left Bank guy", referring to the river Garonne that flows through the Nouvelle-Aquitaine region of France towards Bordeaux. He liked the more tannic Cabernet-Sauvignon-based clarets. He was knowledgeable and could speak with confidence about the gravelly *terroir* with limestone underneath. He could afford the good ones.
>
> He had paid off his attractive home and drove a nearly new BMW. Most of his clothes were tailored and fitted like a glove. You could see he paid attention to grooming and was not shy to indulge in expensive cosmetics for men. Unlike many doctors, he took an array of dietary supplements, almost religiously—an expression of his mortality anxiety. He spoke openly of his fear of serious illness and premature death; he had seen much of it at work. At other times, he spoke of death with an air of resignation about its inevitability.

He wasn't in a relationship, but he was no stranger to romance. His relationships hadn't lasted long except for one from the ages of nineteen to twenty-six. Its traumatic ending accounted for his subsequent reluctance to commit. Other than quite short-term liaisons, he had had an important relationship for nearly two years more recently with Joanne, but he had left in the end. He preferred his own company.

He played the guitar, collected precious gemstones, was fascinated by astronomy—often gazing at the stars through his telescope—and was an avid reader. He liked different genres including self-help, biography, science fiction, and murder mysteries. He played squash competitively but also liked golf which he called "a walk in the park".

He worked in a hospital in the public sector, and strongly believed that he should make his medical skills available to those less fortunate than himself. He had experience in the private sector where he felt more pressured there from the profit-driven commercialisation of medical systems that he found objectionable. "How did medicine ever become a business?" He decried this trend.

He also donated to several charities and felt strongly that society should not allow so many people to be homeless or without food or adequate healthcare. He called the way politicians disregarded the plight of the poorest and most disadvantaged "a national disgrace". He advocated for the first Australians, Aboriginal people, to be acknowledged in the Constitution. At the same time, he held the major political parties in contempt.

Everyone regarded him as "a good person", likeable, easy to be with, agreeable, intelligent, with a quick wit and a sharp sense of humour. His disposition was temperate, not overly happy but far from depressed. Quiet and contained, he could be reserved.

One day, Bradley didn't turn up for work at the hospital. Though this was most unusual, no one thought much of it until he didn't turn up the next day. The police were asked to go around to his house. When they entered his home, they found Bradley dead in his bed. He had taken drugs from the hospital with which he ended his life. He knew exactly how to do it. There was no note.

His friends were baffled and distressed, like my patient, who sobbed on and off during our session. Bradley's one living parent, his father, was shocked, couldn't understand it. His previous partner said there was no sign at all that Bradley was suicidal. It was his decision to separate from her and end their relationship; he was definite about that. He hadn't seemed troubled before this or since. Why had he taken his life?

Meaninglessness

Bradley was not my patient. I had never met him. The information I had was second-hand. All I can do is speculate. Perhaps Bradley had cancer or some fatal disease which he kept to himself. Perhaps he accidentally took an overdose, although this seems unlikely given his medical expertise. Perhaps he had conquered his fear of death and embraced it on his own terms, albeit prematurely. Such musings are the equivalent of reading tea leaves.

This enigmatic case, distressing as it is, leads to a broader field of inquiry. On the "outside", Bradley was successful. What was going on "inside", unavailable to his friends? Note that the account given focuses on the "outside"; any reference to the "inside" is not much more than superficial. Psychotherapists begin to consider the "inside" when people consult us feeling empty or hollow, have no motivation or direction, or when their personal sense of purpose eludes them. Sometimes, they don't want to go on.

Feelings of emptiness, frustration, anxiety, futility, and depression arising from personal history have been called neurotic or an expression of a psychoneurosis. Viktor Frankl termed them "noögenic" (Gk: *νοῦς* = mind + *γένεσις* = origin, becoming) when these feelings arise from existential concerns as a form of spiritual lack. In other words, meaninglessness can be regarded as purely psychological or more of a metaphysical issue. I see no point in separating the two.

Frankl's *Man's Search for Meaning* (2014, originally published in 1959) and his other books *The Will to Meaning, Foundations and Applications of Logotherapy* (1970) and *The Doctor and the Soul: From Psychotherapy to Logotherapy* (1986) are widely read and celebrated. Frankl's approach differs from traditional analytic psychotherapy by focusing on the noögenic origins of suffering with a focus on meaning. Unlike Freud, with whom he associated the will to pleasure, and Adler, with whom he associated the will to power,[12] Frankl's approach was "logotherapy" (Gk: *logos* = meaning). Logotherapy was based on *the will to meaning*. For Frankl, the search for meaning is the primary motivational force for humankind.

While I agree with this emphasis, I question why we would isolate and exclude each of those concepts from the others? Power and pleasure are at the forefront of what causes mental suffering. Here, I bring some of the ideas of logotherapy into psychotherapy in the belief that psychotherapy (and all mental health practices) can be impoverished by the lack of considerations of meaning—and to expand those ideas further. Frankl is concerned with *logos not logic*. For me, logos has its own profound logic and needn't be polarised against logic. (In fact, both words have the same Greek root, *logos*.)

It was Frankl who coined the term "existential vacuum" and characterised it as "a widespread phenomenon of the 20th century". He believed that large numbers of people, perhaps the majority, are at a loss as to the meaning of their lives and their reasons for living. In *Man's Search for Meaning* (2014), he says:

> This is understandable; it may be due to a twofold loss which man has had to undergo since he became a truly human being. At the beginning of human history, man lost some of the basic animal instincts in which an animal's behavior is imbedded and by which

---

[12] In *The Will to Meaning* (1986, p. 41) Frankl associates the will to pleasure with childhood, the will to power with adolescence, and the will to meaning with adulthood, as developmental stages. To me, children seek meaning and power as do adolescents who also seek pleasure!

it is secured … In addition to this, however, man has suffered another loss in his more recent development inasmuch as the traditions which buttressed his behavior are now rapidly diminishing. No instinct tells him what he has to do, and no tradition tells him what he ought to do; sometimes he does not even know what he wishes to do. Instead, he either wishes to do what other people do (conformism) or he does what other people wish him to do (totalitarianism).

Thus, the feelings of emptiness and meaningless have their principal expressions in depression, aggression, and addiction (2014, p. 133). And *Man's Search for Meaning* was first published in German[13] in 1946!

Many instances of suicide could be attributed to this condition but even if not caused by a feeling of meaninglessness,

> it may well be that an individual's impulse to take his life would have been *overcome* had he been aware of some meaning and purpose worth living for. (2014, p. 133, original emphasis)

Was this the case with Bradley? If Bradley had had some meaning and purpose that made life worth living, then surely he would have lived. This seems evident but we cannot trade on assumptions. What is not evident is *why* he didn't have meaning or purpose. It is this *why* that we don't understand—not to be confused by the impressive "exterior", but an "interior" where the *why* is located and where psychotherapy (or logotherapy) might have been able to gain access. There was so much more to Bradley than met the eye.

For Frankl, there is no general answer to the question: *What is the meaning of life?* It is personal, not abstract. Every person must answer this question for themselves in their own way. Apart from the jarring use of "man" and the pronoun "he" to refer to everyone, I like how Frankl addresses this issue:

> As each situation in life represents a challenge to man and presents a problem for him to solve, the question of the meaning of life may actually be reversed. Ultimately, man should not ask what the meaning of his life is, but rather he must recognize that it is *he* who is asked. In a word, each man is questioned by life; and he can only answer to life by *answering for* his own life; to life he can only respond by being responsible. Thus, logotherapy sees in responsibleness the very essence of human existence. (2014, p. 102, original emphasis)[14]

---

[13] The title of the first English translation, published in 1959, was *From Death-Camp to Existentialism*, which is more faithful to the German than the best-known title *Man's Search for Meaning*, also published in 1959.
[14] This calls to mind the work of the twentieth-century philosopher Emmanuel Levinas (1969) and his great work *Totality and Infinity: An Essay on Exteriority*, which, interestingly, was first published (in French) in 1961 shortly after the time the English version of *Man's Search for Meaning* appeared.

Meaning is to be discovered in the world, and not exclusively in oneself as an isolated individual. It is unlikely to be discovered by analysis of your psyche as a closed system. (R. D. Laing, in the 1960s, considered it a mistake of classical psychoanalysis to regard the analysis of an individual psyche as a closed system because the system had to include the person of the analyst—thereby making it a relational system and process.)

Frankl's argument that we, all of us, are responsible (or need to be) points to meaning being discoverable *only* in the world, in society as we find it. It requires going beyond your individual self. He called this "self-transcendence" and referred to giving oneself over to a cause, a creative endeavour, loving another person, and answering the calling that life poses. In addition, Frankl deeply believed that it was essential to realise that unavoidable suffering had meaning, and he attributed his miraculous survival of the Nazi concentration camps, after a long internment, to this attitude.

This, no doubt, influenced his belief that conscience was key in guiding our search to find meaning. Unusually, he defined conscience as "the intuitive capacity to find out the meaning of a situation" (2014, p. 63). Conscience is creative. This follows his belief that the existential vacuum came about because we have become more civilised and socialised, thus losing our animal nature, and, at the same time, traditions and traditional values have become eroded. The danger here is that we become drawn into a deadening mode of conformity—because we have no sense of our own authentic values, direction, and purpose—or subject to totalitarianism. Either we do what other people do—because we don't know what we want to do ourselves—or because we are subject to their will. This is how Frankl arrives at conscience as the driver of the search for meaning and "responsibleness": a response to what is needed and what we are called upon to do.

His uncommon use of the word "conscience" made me think about its meaning. "Con" means "with" or "together". "Science" is derived from the Latin *scire* which means "to know". Conscience is "together with knowledge". When applied to values, this perspective points the way to knowing the difference between right and wrong, or, in a word—ethics. Ethics is constitutive of human relating, and for Frankl conscience is constitutive of the human search for meaning. In this way, finding and creating meaning becomes a relational endeavour.

Filling the void

For Frankl, meaningfulness is found in three main categories: creativity, love/beauty, and suffering. But is meaning simply just "there", waiting to be found? Let's consider how meaning itself *comes into being* (further developed in the next chapter) and the consequences of when it doesn't. We begin with a clinical case involving the existential vacuum.

Clarissa initially consulted me for psychotherapy over two years, commencing at age twenty-seven. She had previously consulted three psychologists, two counsellors, and one psychiatrist but claimed she had not received much help from any. Our discussions included her obsession with food and destructive behaviours involving drugs, alcohol, and sex with an abusive partner named Daniel. Three years later she consulted me for two sessions and then a further two years later Clarissa returned to ongoing therapy.

Now 2018, Clarissa pleaded by phone "I'm going mental and need help". She was ready to commit to weekly sessions again. This time, by her account, the hole that she carried in herself had become "the black hole". It had become a devouring monster that needed filling in any possible way. Clarissa, now thirty-four years old, was better at restraining her tendencies towards self-destructiveness but the feeling inside had become intense. She was struggling to live with it.

She had split with her boyfriend of three years, Matthew, but they remained best friends. She had made some terrible choices with other men except for one named Paul. One night, after she and Paul consumed five bottles of wine together, she turned nasty. The "monster" came out. She called him every name under the sun, verbally attacked him (for no reason), and then went back to Daniel. After a couple of encounters with Daniel abusing her as before, she realised she didn't want that. She apologised to Paul for the verbal bashing she had given him. He said he understood, alcohol could do that to anyone. He could forgive her but wanted to go slowly with her and see how it went.

Clarissa said she was sobbing every day for no reason. She felt completely empty inside. She discovered the only thing that really helped was yoga. She'd taken it up every day, it made her feel better. But the underlying feeling of a painful hollowness was still there and could get the better of her. That's when she would break down. When she fell apart, she cried inconsolably and felt a "madness" that frightened her. That is what she meant by "going mental" in her phone call to me.

Many people tell a variation of Clarissa's story.

Clarissa told me she swings between feeling proud of her achievements, her independence and self-sufficiency, and hating herself. On the positive side, she can support herself, do good work, her business is successful, and she can pay her way. On the negative side, she feels "like a nut case", and has given herself a medical condition (bleeding from the anus)—probably a consequence of alcohol and substance abuse, and her addiction to men that mistreat her. The self-loathing is far stronger than the positives. I suggested that through her "addiction to men that mistreated her" she positioned a man to take the role of antagonist that she holds against herself. (Later, questions arose as to whether this could be a re-enactment of an abusive childhood relationship.)

She had issues with her appearance, her weight, her body, her relationships, and her moods. To me, she looked fine. She was slim, and her weight was nothing like the issue it had been years ago. If anything, I thought Clarissa looked better as a thirty-four-year-old than as a twenty-seven-year-old. My views mean little here—what matters, is how she sees herself, judges herself, and how she feels about herself.

When we examined her inner dialogue, the judgements and criticisms were ferocious—hostile and vicious in the extreme. I could see no useful purpose they served, and we agreed to work on improving her relation to herself. I don't believe you *have to* love yourself—as is commonly espoused. I do believe that self-love expressed by looking after your physical and mental health is desirable. It is also not so simple as to say "change the narrative" as if she could simply switch to another channel at will.

I had been presented with a clear picture of how Clarissa's hateful relationship to herself was generative of her feeling of emptiness, the void and hollowness that she suffered so painfully. I cannot say in a theoretical way that every person who feels an existential void or emptiness suffers from self-loathing at the same time, or that one causes the other. Theoretically, there is an axis upon which some people seem to pivot between a positive narcissism and a negative sense of themselves. A feeling of emptiness (and loneliness) tends to follow the latter, sometimes with a torrent of hostile judgements against themselves—which, of course, reinforces a negative sense of self.

For Clarissa, this internal dynamic became externalised in the form of "hooking up" sexually with men who mistreated her. This had become eroticised—being mistreated aroused her sexually—to the point of becoming an "addiction". Feeling addicted to mistreatment, in turn, generated further judgements against herself in a self-determining, self-perpetuating, and self-fulfilling spiral of events, internal and external, that recurred over time. There was a conflict in her intra-being (relation with self) that became a conflict in her inter-being (relations with others).

> The correlation between self-loathing
> and the feeling of emptiness is a key insight from the
> experience of the existential vacuum.

A negative and self-critical relation to self is not the only cause of emptiness, nor all there is to the existential vacuum. A deeply complex matter entrenched in the broader culture, it manifests itself differently for each individual. I felt glad Clarissa returned to therapy. I know some may think we have been at it for a long time. To me, Clarissa was nearer to the beginning of therapy than the end. Believing anyone can change their thinking by simply telling them to do so, is a delusion, a professional myth. It does not touch the question of meaning or how lasting change happens.

In our next session, Clarissa told me she had been up until 4 a.m. the night before, with Paul. "Sex?" Yes, it was a typical night for her—drinking until 2 a.m., then sex until they passed out.

I asked how it was for her and about her experience of sex in general. Clarissa said she loved sex, but it was blurry for her. She said she had never had sex without being drunk. "Never!" I asked. "Why? What do you think would happen?" And she answered: "It's too intense for me, the feelings are too strong, I get too passionate and lose myself." Clarissa merged psychologically with her partner(s). She used alcohol as a brake on passion and intensity, and the tendency to disappear into the union with another person. It was numbing and distancing. It enabled her to dissociate.

In an existential sense, Clarissa used alcohol to stay alive, to prevent loss of identity into non-being, to continue to exist, to "function". Not that her actual existence was at stake, rather it was *the feeling of existence as a separate person*, the feeling of being—an ontological issue.

Dissociation, whether induced psychologically or through substances, protects against feelings of unbearable pain, suffering, loss, and other consequences of trauma. The tendency towards merging with another person suggests early developmental deficiency or trauma. However, I am reserving judgement as to the possibility of early trauma for Clarissa as she has no corresponding memories to confirm this view.

R. D. Laing's *The Divided Self* (1960) comes to mind in this context. Written when Laing was aged twenty-eight, *The Divided Self* examines schizoid and schizophrenic experience with remarkable lucidity and insight. The many variations of the oft-repeated expression that "in a mad world, only the mad are sane or insanity is a rational response to an irrational world" originate from this book. The book was embraced by the masses, touching a nerve that reverberated throughout popular culture, widely influencing mental health practices to this day.

The split of a divided self manifests itself in many ways, the most prominent being that between mind and body, or more specifically between self and body, and this in the context of self and others. For Clarissa, we can see from the account of her sexual experience that she cannot be wholly "in" her body; rather, she needs to get "out of it". There is a curious paradox that arises when a person wants to be recognised as the person they truly are, but then finds that possibility "too much". Being recognised becomes threatening, invasive, and frightening.

Merging, a defence against separateness, is triggered. Being recognised risks annihilation—the feeling of being swallowed up, subsumed in another, overwhelmed or, in Laing's term, engulfed. To avoid being known is safer, even if lonelier. Isolation raises questions about the *meaning* of your existence and raises doubts about it—as many have discovered through the Covid-19 pandemic.

> "A ship is always safe ashore but that is not what
> it's built for."
>
> (Albert Einstein)

In schizoid experience, a comprehensive false-self system[15] is generated. The aim is to protect the true self or, more accurately, a sense of oneself as genuine, real, alive, separate, and private.

A hyper-awareness of self and others is required to monitor the situation at all times. Self-consciousness can be critical and punishing. A nagging sense of being judged harshly and continuously is then constant, usually arising from self-judgements when there are no others making judgements. This requires vigilance, if not hypervigilance. The body is like a foreign object, something that is dragged around and either mistreated or dressed-up, sometimes in exaggerated ways, to throw others off "who you really are". A person cannot feel fully alive, whole, with a sense of cohesive unity and of substance, in this mode. At its worst, a vacuum is created of meaninglessness and despair: an existential vacuum.

Laing puts it like this:

> The abundance *there* is longed for, in contrast to the emptiness *here;* yet participation without loss of being is felt to be impossible, and also is not enough, and so the individual must cling to his isolation—his separateness without spontaneous, direct relatedness— because in doing so he is clinging to his identity. His longing is for complete union. But of this very longing he is terrified, because it will be the end of his self. He does not wish for a relationship of mutual enrichment and exchange of give-and-take between two beings "congenial" to each other. (1965, pp. 91–92, original emphasis)

Well, "he" does wish for it, but "he" must be secure in "his" separateness to manage such a relationship without risk of loss of self. So, this separateness is a disconnectedness.

Elaborating on the quote above: *Separateness without spontaneous, direct relatedness to another person is the beginning of the descent into meaninglessness and isolation in an existential vacuum.*

There is a rich ambiguity in the word "separateness". In one sense, it is necessary for con-nectedness to be possible. In another sense, you can be too separate to the point of being cut off from others.

---

[15] Laing told me Winnicott was cross that he didn't give Winnicott a footnote when he wrote about the false self in his first book. Laing rebutted Winnicott saying that references to false self were abundant elsewhere in psycho-analysis and especially in philosophy, in Kierkegaard, Sartre, and Heidegger, for example.

Some of the above applied to Clarissa but not all. She wanted to be loved, but she didn't know what love was and wasn't sure she was ready. When she was loved by someone who treated her respectfully and with care, she felt bored. She was more excited by mistreatment and abuse.

Now Clarissa sobs every day "for no reason". She feels completely empty inside, a painful hollowness. Nothing is happening or being done to her to make her sob—there is no reason in the present. But nothing happening *means* something. How she feels *is* a reason to sob. Presumably, her feelings are welling up from the past and expressing ungrieved losses and unprocessed traumas.

The disembodiment of the mind–body split—for Clarissa, anaesthetising herself with alcohol, numbing the body to make sex less intense—removes the body from experience. Her "self" is removed, she is hardly there. Without her body at the centre of her emotional life, she is lost.

> ## Cut off from your body, you become no-body.

As Laing says, embodiment is no insurance policy against an apparent lack of meaning—but it is a good start. To be nobody, not "a person", empty and hollow, is a common basis for depression and anxiety, especially social anxiety. Many people feel uncomfortable in social situations, under pressure to be something they're not, or to perform according to a role they don't want, or feel doesn't fit. Some pretend to be engaged by conversations or make positive noises to others they don't really mean or feel—then become self-conscious due to a sense of acting falsely. Will it be noticed?

One of the consequences of self-consciousness, beyond hyper-awareness of being seen, is a fear of being *seen through*. The feeling is one of transparency, as if you were made of glass. This is also an element of Imposter Syndrome in which a person feels afraid that others will see through them and realise they are not up to their role or status or responsibility. *You are not who you are cracked up to be.* Imposters are not deserving of the credit they have been given. It is a matter of time before they are found out and fall. The feeling is independent of the facts, but the fear of falling or failing is intense, as is the fear of being seen to fall.

Often, it turns out that all the fears of others' critical judgements are projections of one's own reflected back imaginatively. You fear others realising the "truth" about you from your own negative point of view.

> ## The anxiety of social anxiety is as much about being found as it is about being found out.

Social anxiety and self-consciousness go together. In both cases, there may be a feeling of playing a role or wearing a mask. Some people feel they are always wearing a mask. After *The Divided Self* (1965) was published, there were debates as to whether it was ever possible *not* to wear a mask or play a role. *Is a truly authentic way of being even possible?*

Part of the false-self system is playing at being yourself such that nothing really matters, no one can ever affect you, or hurt you, because no one can ever really know you or get close enough. (Bradley?) Again, nothing *means* something. This may not stop you from having relationships, sexual experiences, doing a job, or becoming established in a career. You can get married, have children, friendships, and colleagues. One of Laing's patients said: "I have been married for many years and made love with my wife many times. But I have never really made love with my wife at all because I wasn't really there." She didn't know.

> In the absence of a spontaneous natural, creative, relationship with the world which is free from anxiety, the "inner self" thus develops an overall sense of inner impoverishment, which is expressed in complaints of the emptiness, deadness, coldness, dryness, impotence, desolation, worthlessness, of the inner life … phenomenologically, we are justified in speaking of the vacuum that the self feels itself to be. (1965, pp. 90–91)

If you have made yourself, in a sense, unreal, then everything that transpires between this unreal self and the world is going to feel that it lacks *meaning* and *purpose*. This is why psychotherapy needs to promote the development of an authentic sense of self.

The experience of emptiness varies greatly. There are countless talks, texts, and discussions about the meaning of emptiness, especially in Buddhism. There it has a positive quality, a state of sufficiency, reached through meditation, and the unravelling of desire and striving. Yet for many, it is one of the worst feelings there is. I think the term "emptiness" can refer to different states of being and have different meanings. In the Buddhist sense, there is a feeling of sufficiency that does not depend on *having* anything in particular. You are as you are, and there is nothing you need beyond what is available to you. The world has possibilities and limitations that remain unquestioned. The associated feeling is acceptance and satisfaction, nothing else is required to be okay.[16]

However, the feeling of emptiness discussed here is practically opposite. It is a feeling that *nothing* can fill or satisfy. There is a longing for *something*, a need to overcome a sense of incompleteness, or insufficiency—to fill a painful hollowness. A great deal is needed to fill this hole though it isn't clear what it would take. It is an existential vacuum. To turn this state into the Buddhist sense of sufficiency would involve a 180-degree shift in experience. This is more than a change of attitude; it would amount to experiencing the world and oneself in it completely differently.

---

[16] My friend Ross Bolleter, himself a Zen Roshi, tells me that he understands the Dalai Lama to have said what shocked Tibetans most about Westerners was their degree of self-loathing.

When a person feels empty, they may well be impelled to (try to) fill themselves up with something to overturn that feeling. Filling up with food is an obvious one. Nowadays, obesity and what is called "diabesity" (diabetes + obesity) exists in epidemic proportions. Or fill up with money, sex, alcohol, or drugs, shopping, adventures, and technology—how many people are addicted to their phones? Notice the quality of chasing something, of pursuit, of grasping, and of accumulating—the idea of the life to come.[17] Most of us seem to be always trying to get somewhere. Even with the endless scrolling of smartphones, tablets, and computers there is a sense of searching, trying to discover something, or uncover—the real news, not the fake news, how can we know? We surf more and more webpages; we're hypnotised by them. Filling up doesn't work though; it isn't fulfilling, it lacks meaning. The Buddha's principal insight was exactly that this chasing after something and trying to grab and hold onto it is the source of suffering. He called it "desire". Desire is a complex phenomenon in a modern social context. Desire is the fuel that drives many of us.

The Buddha wandered around 500 years before Christ and had it worked out well. He had been a Prince, people respected him, cared for him, fed him. He had no need of money. He didn't really need anything. He could meditate, reflect, give talks, and disseminate wisdom. There is still a lot to be said for wandering, and a lot to be said for wondering.

Contemporary living makes tremendous demands on most of us too, that didn't exist in the time of the Buddha. I'm sure there were other sorts of demands then, not least surviving. Survival remains a struggle for many today, though the meaning of *survival* also has quite a different complexion now. Requirements and threats to survival exist not just in the context of your bodily health, but also in your relation to yourself and others, in addition to the genetic, constitutional, environmental factors and, of course—lifestyle. For occupational health, often your relationships with others in your workplace have as much, if not more, to do with your *health* as your work performance. Financial health is a battle for many people in a world where living is increasingly expensive, being scammed or stolen-from more commonplace, and the rules can change without your even knowing. Add credit, debt, un(der)employment, and the volatility of financial markets (not least crypto!) and you have a formula for financial ill-health.

Is this preoccupation with health healthy? Is there a risk in becoming overly preoccupied with health?[18]

> "Attention to health is life's greatest hindrance."
>
> (Plato)

---

[17] This is a reference to Samuel Beckett's famous play *Endgame* and this poignant exchange: "Clov: 'Do you believe in the life to come?' Hamm: 'Mine was always that.'"

[18] Written before the 2020 pandemic.

I believe the opposite. However, it is worth thinking about ways that you can become too pre-occupied with health issues: what ingredients are in the food you eat, have you done enough exercise, is your sleep quality and quantity good enough, is weight a persistent issue, body image, and so on? Are there bodily symptoms or sensations that worry you? Do you fear cancer (or something) is right around the corner? Has your life become dominated by an illness or disability and its treatment? Are we, as a culture, overdoing it to our detriment? Over-worrying about health can be a source of mental ill-health. There is a freedom from worry that is healthier than obsessing. No doubt there is a balance between being health-aware and not going overboard about it. Hyper-awareness can be a hindrance and is no better than a lack of awareness.

"There is more wisdom in your body than in your deepest philosophy." Friedrich Nietzsche's quote points to listening to what your body tells you of your health needs more than trying to keep up with the endless theories, dogmas, "hacks", and philosophies on how to live for health. The individual focus on "health" as a subject can take you away from your relation to your body and your relation to other people, to be left wandering anxiously in the labyrinth of your mind. This is not the territory of a practice of healthy living and mental well-being.

The Vietnamese Buddhist monk and peace activist Thich Nhat Hanh coined the term "inter-being" to refer to the way that our *being* is essentially with others. We are not isolates. When people feel empty in the colloquial sense, there is probably some sense of disconnected-ness that has occurred, or maybe has always been the case. Disconnectedness is disconnected from something or someone, from others; there must be an other from whom you are disconnected. Or could it be that a person can also be disconnected within, disconnected from self? Perhaps we should also speak of *intra-being*, which means being at one with self, integrated, together.

Generally, we can be in harmony with ourselves or fall out with ourselves. We can be in conflict inside, or we can be resolved. We can be whole and wholesome or split and divided. At odds. At a loose end. At sea. It is harder to be connected to an other when you are not connected to yourself. What does this mean? It is odd to speak of being connected to self; it implies the self is two things that are connected to each other. What kind of wholeness could that be?

Yet, consciousness does involve an *inner* dialogue. There is a curious sort of conversation going on in the privacy of yourself most of the time. Who are you speaking to? Who is the speaker? Who is the listener? What sorts of communications are you making to yourself? Are they supportive and encouraging or are they critical and undermining? Some people speak to themselves more harshly than they would to their worst enemy. Are you your own worst enemy? A divided self? Could this have something to do with the feeling of emptiness? The existential vacuum? The sense of a lack of meaning?

In therapy, Clarissa accessed a deep well of feelings regarding the loss of Adrian, her first love at age fourteen, that she had never been able to process before. Shortly after they made love for the first time, he killed himself. This was an immensely complex and powerful relationship at a time of life when young teens typically feel their feelings intensely. Clarissa was deeply in love with Adrian, she has never felt love for a partner as strongly since, she told me. Adrian used heroin and was also dating another girl. Clarissa had sex with him that was voluntary and consensual. Is having "full sex" so young necessarily traumatic? (Clarissa didn't think so).

What constitutes a trauma? One of Adrian's last communications was to tell his brother to tell Clarissa he loved her. Then he hanged himself. Clarissa went from a feeling of being deeply in love to one of overwhelming, unbearable loss. How could she process this traumatic loss with her emotional capacities, as far as they had developed then? She couldn't. Could she do that now, with me? It is hard to say exactly what "fully processed" means; it's complicated. For Clarissa in her thirties, "Adrian" is a distant memory. The idea of "Adrian" is a mental object, an object or concept of mind for Clarissa. This can change with the passage of time and has changed. Processing involves what Adrian meant to Clarissa then and how the idea of Adrian has evolved in her mind.

The felt pain of loss is woven through every step and stage. The process of grieving is both cognitive and emotional; indeed, to be "full" involves the integration of the two while connecting with their "object" of loss. The inability to process this loss sufficiently is an obstacle preventing her relationships from becoming as meaningful as they could otherwise be. Closeness is too dangerous; it means either merging with the other or keeping them out, at a distance. While this explains a lot, issues of the existential vacuum, emptiness, meaninglessness, relationship shortcomings, and bodily symptoms are profoundly complex and not reducible to simple psychological explanations or, in this case, not being able to process grief due to developmental limitations.

What is the point of going through all that emotional pain now? Going through it moves us on and frees up energy and emotional capacities for new possibilities in the present. Some losses are never put behind us completely. However, the integration of the past into the living field of experience in the present is indispensable for meaning to take the place of nothingness. The movement of a psychotherapeutic process is from

- the mental to the develop-mental
- cognitive to felt
- abstract to real
- conceptual to lived.

More than *a problem*, the existential vacuum of meaning detailed in Clarissa's case is a deeply embedded cultural pattern of experience and behaviour that pertains to many people in different ways. Is there anyone who cannot identify with some aspect of Clarissa's feelings of emptiness or a lack of meaning or purpose at some point in their life? I am all too aware of those tendencies in myself.

You can feel the consequences of the existential vacuum without having a diagnosable mental disorder that requires medication. Numbing pain or avoiding suffering through medications or psychological techniques is already part of the problem and not the solution to it.

It is easy to get caught up in the drive to diagnose. The existential vacuum does bring many *symptoms* of a mental disorder in its wake. Even if treatment is successful in making you feel better, and often it isn't, the underlying issues remain, the object of your suffering is kept at a distance, abstracted, and deferred.

It is a matter of time before what is underlying becomes overbearing and cannot be deferred any longer. Medication and positive psychology are strategies of postponement. Some things cannot be postponed indefinitely. Postponement sustains disorder rather than resolves it.

> When what is underlying is unbearable,
> it becomes unavoidable.

Effective therapy helps patients find and create meaning in their lives. And the question of what makes life worth living is addressed in the process. Feeling better, happier, finding more purpose and direction, feeling that life is fulfilling and satisfying are natural outcomes without having to resort to synthetic or artificial means. Then, you don't have to make anything—the life to come—other than what it is. Rather you can live the life you are given, meaning-fully.

Most of the issues for Clarissa, and for the great majority of us, arise from childhood, family-of-origin issues, and early relationship dynamics. Effective therapy cannot give you another childhood. Understanding something of early childhood development, however, sheds enormous light on what does need to happen in the present to promote emotional development in the service of overcoming issues of the existential vacuum and developing more of a sense of self. The implications for living are profound. We need to begin at the earliest determination of meaning, thus returning to the question in the opening of this section: How does meaning *come into being*? We address this question in the next chapter.

The developmental tilt

My frequent use of the metaphor of development requires further comment. In a seminal paper by Stephen A. Mitchell—one of the founders of the relational movement in psychoanalysis and psychotherapy—"Object relations theories and the developmental tilt" (1984), he argues that the reliance on development skews psychoanalytic theory and has consequences.

As much as I value Mitchell's work and am largely aligned with the relational movement, I disagree. Mitchell dichotomises the use of the developmental perspective as either correcting the deficiencies of childhood development or providing a new and positive adult experience of intimacy and connection in the experience of therapy. It is both, as I see it. I see more benefit than consequence in the developmental tilt, of which this book is an example. My experience of therapy and of therapy practice has proven to me that we should not be shy of the developmental tilt.

After finishing the manuscript for this book, I discovered a journal article by Steven H. Cooper that also offers a critique of Mitchell's position on the developmental tilt. He says:

> Mitchell's critique of the developmental tilt may have also steered us away from the intrinsic developmental components in the psychoanalytic process. (2021, p. 367)

Cooper pays homage to Mitchell but claims his position on the developmental perspective is too reductionistic, as I say above. We will go on to discuss Winnicott's ideas in greater detail from here. Cooper says that Winnicott's view of interpretation was more about giving patients an experience of becoming themselves—especially through an experience of play—than using interpretation to impart information, insight, explanation, and understanding, as in more traditional, epistemological approaches to therapy (2021). For me, it is both, as neither cancels the value of the other.

> Winnicott's use of play as the center of the analytic process created early forms of ontological psychoanalysis. (2021, p. 367)

And he concludes his article:

> Unfortunately, by minimizing the existential and ontological elements of Winnicott's revolutionary contributions, we have perhaps not fully utilized the benefits of a marriage of "talking about what is going on here" (Levenson, 1972, 1983) with "helping patients to be" (Cooper, under review). (2021, p. 368)

And that is exactly what this book is about.

CHAPTER 4

The origin of the capacity for meaning-making

The transitional experience of the small child
may be the basis of everything else.
D. W. Winnicott

Having identified the existential vacuum as a major area of neglect in mental health, we first need to find our way into the world of the small child to address the question of how meaning comes into being. I start by looking at the earliest experience of an object becoming meaningful to a small child.

It is not possible to locate the very first object of meaning with any certainty, but it is possible to see the first *sign* of such an object when a child begins to develop a relationship to *something* and becomes attached to it. Winnicott calls this a "transitional object". The classic example of a transitional object is the teddy bear; children are attached to their teddies or whatever object much of the time, and especially when going to sleep.

Why "transitional"? What does this term refer to? Transitioning from what, to what, and why is it important? Winnicott calls the transitional object the child's first "not-me possession". It doesn't have to be a teddy bear. It is often a stuffed animal or a blanket or piece of material. Not every child has one but when they do, it is obvious. It is noticeable how important such an object can be to a child; it *means* something.

The expression "not-me possession" refers to forming a relationship with an object that is separate.

> You cannot see it (an object as separate)
> if you *be* it (are merged with it).

A relationship with an object as separate from self is a developmental advance from early relationships that are described as fused or merged. In very early development, objects such as mother's breast are understood to be experienced as an extension of the child, as if a part of the child or belonging to the child. The beginnings of an experience of separation of self from objects in the world marks the origin of the possibility of a relationship in a true sense: an involvement between two reasonably separate entities. Here, we mark an essential step in the capacity for meaning-making.

"Separation" begins to indicate what the term "transitional" refers to: the transition from fused to separate, although these positions are not absolute. Terms like "fused" and "separate" describe ways of experiencing, they are psychological tendencies, not a purely physical position in time and space. The transitional object can be seen as an extension of the child in the process of developing a relationship with a separate entity. The uses of such an object can be manifold: to relieve anxiety, to self-soothe, to assert control, ownership, or possession, and even to give love.

If you think this is only a discussion about childhood experience, consider the above applied to adult uses of mobile (cell) phones. Could our phones be the new transitional objects of adulthood? Phones are interesting in this regard as they are used both to separate and to connect.

Transition is born out of fusion

The way we, all of us, experience the world in terms of fusion and separateness has everything to do with emptiness or meaning-fullness in living—as evidenced in Clarissa's experience.

Many children who lack a transitional object are still developing normally and creating a basis for meaningful living. Transitional objects simply enable us to see something of this process as it is unfolding. Without a visible object, the process is hidden from view. It may well be occurring *normally*, but privately, and may be imperceptible to others.

The child adopts an object of their own choosing. They become attached to it, sometimes they are inseparable from it. Questions arise—*How does the transitional object become an object of meaning for the child?* Why this object? How is meaning found here and not there—or is it created? Winnicott asks us not to resolve these questions though there is a value in examining them (1971, p. 1).[19]

---

[19] The first reference to transitional objects appears in Winnicott's 1951 essay "Transitional Objects and Transitional Phenomena", which becomes Chapter 1 of *Playing and Reality* (1971).

The first meaningful object holds clues to the origins of the capacity for meaning-making; at least as far as we can see.

> # Meaning gives value to living.

As adults, it is essential to value *something*—this can include a person, an activity, a cause, work, raising children, a creative endeavour, or serving a higher power. However, are you fused with your "object of meaning" or are you separate? How you invest yourself makes all the difference between meaningful, functional activities and those that become harmful. (Could you live without your phone, for example, for a day, a week, forever?)

> Steph was twenty-five years old when she first consulted me. She was in crisis. Her fiancé of four years, Jake, had left her; he not only left her but left town as well. He said he wasn't ready to be tied down for life. He loved her but couldn't keep going in the relationship. He wanted to travel, see the world, experience other relationships; he said he needed "to find himself".
>
> Steph was shocked. They were engaged to marry. She thought she'd found "the one", and all she wanted was to be with him. Her idea of her future was all laid out in her mind and had been for some years. She saw children, a modest but comfortable home, and a life partner to have fun and share everything with. His change of heart "killed" her.
>
> When she arrived at my office for her first consultation, she was suicidal. She had been quite broken down, she told me, but she was more composed now. She didn't want to go on, she was clear about that. Her life was over. There was no point.

I've heard many, many people speak like this, and I've heard many people express a *feeling* of not wanting to go on. I had never heard anyone speak as Steph did. Hard to describe: there was a coldness, a definiteness, a sense of resignation about it. I felt one hundred per cent certain that I would never see her again if I let her leave my office. But I couldn't exactly take her hostage.

> I spent most of the consultation trying to figure out what to do. I had been running psychotherapy trainings and there was a class underway in the seminar room across the hallway. I recalled that a colleague, RW, a psychiatrist, was attending the class. I asked Steph to hold on at the end of the session and asked her permission to discuss what we'd spoken of and to bring someone else in. She agreed.
>
> In front of Steph, I described the situation to RW, and together we agreed there was no question Steph needed to be in hospital. With a bit of convincing, together we

persuaded Steph to accept a place at a private hospital nearby, after determining no public facilities were available.

I was afraid to let Steph out of my sight and with her consent, I drove her there myself. It can be difficult to know the difference between a countertransference[20] enactment and a duty of care that involves a life-saving intervention. Suddenly, I remembered the words of R. D. Laing in one supervision session decades earlier: "If you elect to get out of your chair to 'do something', you should consider very carefully if you are acting-out without realising it." Acting-out or not, I took Steph to the hospital and sat with her through her psychiatric intake interview. I was afraid to leave.

Things became more bizarre from there. Halfway through, the admitting psychiatrist asked her if she had health insurance and Steph said *no*. Despite her mental state, the psychiatrist stood up, said the interview was over; she couldn't stay there. I reacted angrily and protested. I argued with the psychiatrist[21] and we arrived at a compromise: I put $1,100 on my credit card (acting-out?)[22] to cover the cost of two nights, in advance, for Steph to remain at the hospital. This would also provide time to engage Steph's parents to cover the cost of a longer stay. Once Steph's admission was secured, I immediately phoned her parents and pleaded with them to pay for the remaining twelve days required to keep Steph safe, and to recover the deposit I had already paid.

Her parents refused. They said she was independent and would have to work it out for herself. I countered but they became more resistant. In the end, I resorted to my worst tactics of guilting and shaming: "It is my professional opinion that you will never see your daughter again if you do not support her in hospital at this time. If you can live with that, then that is your business, but I believe you will regret it. She can be helped but it will take a little time and a bit of your money."

They paid. Steph got looked after and medicated for two weeks. And I met with her for sessions at the hospital over this period. Despite my criticisms of psychiatry, such interventions can be necessary.

At the end of the two weeks, Steph felt she could carry on and informed me that she had an offer from a cousin to stay on the family's farm in a beautiful place in remote countryside. She felt that was just what she needed. I was apprehensive of her being isolated but certainly staying in town was only reminding her of her life with Jake and the loss of it.

---

[20] Countertransference is a technical term in psychoanalysis and psychotherapy that has different meanings and usages. Sometimes, countertransference is a valuable source of information and often a source for interpretation rather than action. Here, it refers to my acting *instead of* interpreting.

[21] Here, we have the juxtaposition of two psychiatrists, one who cares (RW) and goes above and beyond and one who is only concerned about his fee. This is what I mean by "psychiatry is not a unified field".

[22] Such heroics are not a normal part of psychotherapy practice.

We had some phone sessions. After a couple of months there, Steph's whole disposition changed. She gradually grew to feel more positive. She was no longer overwhelmed by grief, loss, and hopelessness about the future. She was offered a job on the farm, and it sounded like she was starting to have fun.

She loved living in the country and discovered she had a passion for animal husbandry, and for growing vegetables. They went to town every week and sold their produce at a farmer's market where she grew to feel part of a community. Steph had discovered a way of living that worked for her. And her former suicidality evaporated, to my profound relief.[23]

This is not the only time I have had to put a patient in hospital and, also, not the only time I've driven one there in my car. I am thankful for the hospital and medical staff despite the initial roadblock about finance. "Professional" means privileging the interest of patients, especially when financial interests compete with patients' needs.

Therapists also tolerate and manage much anxiety about potential harm when it seems imminent for patients. Most of the time we rationalise: this danger belongs to this person's life, and I cannot go home with them and protect them. I can only discuss issues in consultations and hope that makes enough of a difference. There is a limit to what therapy can offer but we also have to live with the outcome. Choices as to how far to go beyond sessional contact to express care are amongst the most difficult therapists make. Boundaries are essential, so is duty of care. There exists a tension between remaining in the professional frame and looking after the needs of patients, especially when those needs become extreme.

Steph's attachment to Jake was more of a fusion than an attachment to a transitional object, much less to a "separate object". When she lost the relationship, it was as if her life support had been withdrawn. She could see no future. She had lost her *self*. And she was about to lose her life completely—that's how it looked to me. Anyone who has experienced the pain of an unexpected break-up knows how agonising, and even disintegrating, it can be. For Steph, being left by her fiancé, her ultimate life partner, was traumatising. It was not only the loss of a relationship but also the loss of her dream of the future. This dream served as fuel for living; without it, her ability to go-on-being was called into question (an example of both an ontological and existential issue).

Life has a way of throwing unexpected losses at us. It's hard, if not impossible, to prepare for them. The *can't live without it* quality has a sense of fusion. It would be tragic if you lose your life because of a loss you couldn't have anticipated. In that case, the loss of the "object"

---

[23] This occurred during 1993/1994. I hadn't heard from Steph since then but amazingly, one week after I wrote this story some twenty-four years later, she contacted me and came up to Perth from the country with her partner of ten years to consult me on an altogether different matter. They had three children and had been living happily. Now, in her late forties, she's having regular sessions with me again, which has continued intermittently for over three years since. Talk about synchronicity!

equates to a loss of self. It turns the loss of something, or someone valued, into a global loss of everything. This is a risk when someone means the world to you.

In this story, perhaps Steph found and created for herself a transitional experience through living on her cousin's family's farm. Here, the transitional "object" was a whole way of living rather than an object in the sense of a person or "thing". Living on the farm functioned like the teddy to a small child. I don't mean to diminish the experience for Steph; I am trying to make comprehensible the function of transitional objects.

The transition is from a cut-off, isolated, interior space in yourself—often a space that is "dark" and desolate, a dead space—to a connected space of involvement with other people, one that includes meaningful activities, and possibilities for taking pleasure in living. It can also include a role for yourself, such as Steph found on the farm, and a place in a community where you feel a sense of belonging. This is not exactly a move from inner to outer. Rather, it is a move from cut-off to more connected, from withdrawn to involved with others.

Where a capacity for meaningful living exists, there is no need for an analysis of how or why you become invested in the "objects" of your life. Life isn't perfect or complete, there is always some lack. Okay, live with that. Where there is suffering, then a reflective analysis is called for in yourself and, if wanted, in a formal professional sense. Indeed, it is beneficial if that process, intra-personal or interpersonal, discovers where meaning has been lost and how it can be recovered or renewed afresh. Losses must be processed and grieved, as therapists help their clients move on. Otherwise, depression prevails, often accompanied by its close cousin, anxiety.

> Therapy relieves suffering by enabling it
> to be gone through.

With Steph, my primary aim was to keep her alive long enough for her outlook to improve.

Transition means separation

In questioning how meaning originates, we need to understand transitionality, and for that to make any sense, we need to know what comes before and after a transition. Developmentally speaking, fusion, also called merging, comes first. Steph's story above and Clarissa's from the previous chapter, are examples. After merging, a balance needs to be developed between transitional experiencing and a sense of separateness. Maturity could be a name for that balance. Maybe what comes after maturity is enlightenment, but I cannot speak for that.

When I speak of fusion, I am referring to an experience through which the boundary between self and other feels porous. Much of your psychological experience, that is *the way you experience the world*, is coloured by the degree of separateness or union you feel with significant others. Experience begins with biology and environment; no one can fully separate them (though many have tried). Each informs the other. There is no biology without a conducive environment, and there is no environment without a viable biology.

Biologically, fusion begins at conception. Two "things" come together, sperm and egg, to form a zygote. In simple terms, two come together to form one. But even after implantation, this one—now in the embryonic phase—is still "in" another, the mother. The embryo grows (for about eleven weeks) to become a human foetus. This growth involves a division of cells while remaining implanted in the uterus. The foetus is literally tied to the placenta during its intra-uterine life.

Notice the structure of fusion, two (a twosome or couple) becomes one, the one is implanted in and enveloped by another while tied to its life support (a twosome within one, a dual unity).[24]

Baby is born, the cord is cut, baby goes from "in" to "out", from "in" the bodily environment of mother to "out" and "in" the worldly environment, an environment still mainly defined by the primary carer(s). Even after birth, there remains a continuity with the body of the mother if she breastfeeds. Where does her body end and baby's begin? What is "me" and what is "not me"? Think of the flow of breast milk in this light: at what point does what belongs to mother belong to baby?—also an analogue for the umbilical cord.

The demarcation of separateness is not clear. Babies cannot survive on their own, they are one hundred per cent dependent—a merger, also a dual unity, is now purely psychological. This quality of dependency qualifies the experience of fusion and becomes co-dependency if shared by both parties. Jake evidently did not share in a co-dependency. *Only Steph could not live without Jake.*

I would surmise that Steph's fused state led him to *have to* leave. Such a high level of emotional dependency is burdensome. This is the same type of burden children feel when a parent is so fused with their parental role, they cannot let go and allow the child to separate as an emerging young adult. Steph had not yet achieved a balance of being a separate, individual person in her own psychology, and, as such, a member of a couple relationship. She was so "in" it, she was immersed and enveloped (like a foetus?), so invested that without the relationship *it felt like* there was nothing left of her. She was metaphorically destroyed by Jake leaving; the only thing left was to finish herself off concretely.

Embryologically and experientially, there is a transition from intra-uterine experience, through birth, to becoming a separate, individual person. There is a transition from being tied to the umbilical cord and attached to the placenta, from being immersed in amniotic fluid and enveloped by the womb, to being whole and separate from mother's body. The metaphors of our earliest experience, both pre- and post-natal, are what need to be negotiated through the process of transitional experiencing later in life—being tied or attached, immersed, enveloped,

---

[24] By dual unity, I mean there is the unity of foetus and placenta within the uterus, and the unity of the whole intra-uterine "package" within the body of the mother.

supported, held, contained, nourished, and *connected*—these terms describe not only growing up but continue to apply to later adult experience in relationships. Indeed, such words are the common currency describing the dynamics of adult exchanges.

> Steph's relationship with Jake had become like a womb, a container, a vehicle. She was enfolded within the relationship, all that it meant to her and her dreams of the future. Without it, her support system collapsed. Her will to live evaporated and her suffering was overwhelming. Once the attachment was cut through by Jake's abrupt leaving, it was *as if* the placenta stopped feeding her. She still loved him but there was nothing coming back. All she could think to do was end her life. It was *as if* he had pulled the plug on her life support. She felt her life had ended.
> Being thrust out of the relationship, expelled from the container of the womb, was like a premature birth that risked being a stillbirth.
> Steph was beyond grieving. To grieve requires a sense of separateness from the object or person that has been lost. Grief applies to the loss of something other. Her disposition of cold, steely resolve was so alarming to me partly because it was so far from a more usual expression of grief.

In one way of looking at it, her suffering was exacerbated because she identified fully with being *in* something, a present and future relationship with Jake. When she was cast *out* of it, by him leaving, she felt abandoned and more so—annihilated.

Of course, if she had little reaction to Jake leaving, if she had said "Oh well, that's too bad, I'll just have to go out and get another boyfriend", this would also be questionable. If she had registered little sense of loss or grief and said "No problem, Jake, you go find yourself—have a great life—I'll be fine, being single again could be fun", as a therapist I would have to ask: "Really?" While being separated and hence, separate, might be manageable, that doesn't mean there shouldn't be a painful sense of loss and grief, a need to mourn in the service of moving on. Such a radical change is bound to hurt and be challenging, to say the least.

> The loss of your fused object can feel like a death.

*   *   *

Babies and small children are forever putting things in their mouths, rubbing their upper lip, stroking, clutching, cuddling their special objects, and clearly using them for soothing and to reduce anxiety or fear. If put down to sleep on their own in a darkened room, a transitional object may be the only sleeping pill that works to settle a baby. Teddies reduce tension and distress; there is pain involved in growing into a separate person. There are many possible feelings arising for children of all ages (and for adults) at moments of separateness and aloneness. They range from feeling a little unsettled to painfully disconnected to inconsolable grief or fear. *Where's my mum?*—this environment that once held me.

In one moment, a transitional object can be forgotten, and baby can get interested in something else. In another moment, it is a lifesaver. It is the indispensable saviour that keeps baby from panic, and unbearable distress. At any age, adults are at risk of slipping into despair, depression, anxiety, obsessive rumination, or some other mental "condition" without something that helps keep their heads above water as the transitional object does for a baby.

Without any support, everyday experience can swing from a little uneasy to desperate, and then follows the question: *Why go on?* I'm not saying adults need teddies, rather adults need something meaningful that functions the way teddies do for the small child.

> Meaning, or lack of it,
> is a defining quality of your self and life.

The "paradox" of meaning-making

For Frankl, meaning is discovered in the world, and not invented. Winnicott discusses meaning differently and has a different perspective on how we should approach the question of where meaning comes from. He explains that the origin of a capacity to find or create meaning involves a "paradox":

> It is now generally recognised, I believe, that what I am referring to in this part of my work is not the cloth or the teddy bear that the baby uses—not so much the object used as the use of the object. I am drawing attention to the *paradox* involved in the use by the infant of what I have called the transitional object. My contribution is to ask for a paradox to be accepted and tolerated and respected, and for it not to be resolved. By flight to split-off intellectual functioning it is possible to resolve the paradox, but the price of this is the loss of the value of the paradox itself.
>
> This paradox, once accepted and tolerated, has value for every human individual who is not only alive and living in this world but is also capable of being infinitely enriched by exploitation of the cultural link with the past and with the future. (1971, pp. xi–xii, original emphasis)

It is a difficult and complex statement. Winnicott asks for the paradox not to be resolved, but a true paradox cannot be resolved. He doesn't say what the paradox is here, his reference to it is oblique. As I understand it, Winnicott sees a paradox in whether the meaning the transitional object holds for the child comes from the object itself or from the child. I'm not sure this is a paradox. I agree it is important not to answer this question, that something is lost in resolving it—if it can be resolved.

"Not so much the object used but the use of the object"—this is an important distinction. The most important thing is not what baby chooses or what you or I or the clients above choose as their most meaningful object, but how it is used.

Every human individual is capable of being infinitely (!) enriched by exploitation of the cultural link with the past and with the future. What does this mean? Infinite is without limit. Fancy being enriched without limit. How? You exploit a cultural link with the past by claiming your history, by knowing where you've come from, your cultural origins, as far as you can ever know. *Those who don't learn from the past are doomed to repeat it!* This links to the future by building something, something that has meaning in the context of the past. It doesn't have to be a physical structure, but it is likely to be structured. You can build a relationship or a family. You can build a company. You can build a fortune. Or you can build a portfolio of positive experiences. You don't have to build a thing, you can build a life that is meaningful for yourself and, also for others, too. You can build a way of living that works.

What matters is for *something* to mean *something* to you and for you to mean *something* to *someone*. It is not important to explain why—that is split-off intellectual[25] functioning. Rather, it is more important to dismantle and remove the reasons *why not*, when meaning is not happening or completely missing. Then, we need to build the right conditions for the emergence of meaning if that hasn't already happened through your early experience and development. That is how psychotherapy should proceed to be developmental later for adults.

For the small child who adopts a transitional object, something can be seen to mean something perhaps for the very first time, at the child's own initiation. The notion of transitional object involves the initiation of the capacity for symbolic experience. The use of an object in this way signifies the origins of symbol formation, a process that is notably lacking in the adult who cannot find or create meaning anywhere.

The term "symbolic" means that one thing stands for another. Teddy *is* the child's most prized possession. Claiming it, owning it, endowing it with value—is what makes it symbolic— it makes more of it than it is, in itself. It is the meaning of the teddy (or whatever object) that makes it a symbol. The process of symbol formation is a function of the inner life and becomes

---

[25] Many people suffer from "over-thinking"—I hear about it in sessions. Over-thinking or over-analysing is a person's attempt to work something out, but they don't know how to think in a way that reaches to insight and understanding, and implications for acting differently, more effectively. Instead, they go over this issue again and again. Thinking works best when it is not "split-off", in other words, when it is connected to how you feel, to your history and present culture and to relevant others. Besides, not everything can be figured out by thinking.

a source for symbolisation later, the formulating into an expressive language to communicate what is meaningful.

> Symbolisation, the use of language to convey what is meaningful, is the heart of psychotherapy, and development, too.

The value of processing in the inner life is preserved by not being challenged, as Winnicott indicates:

> it shall exist as a resting place for the individual engaged in the perpetual human task of keeping inner and outer reality separate yet interrelated. (1971, p. 2)

Presumably, Winnicott means we all need a rest from the task of processing. But meaning-making does not depend upon keeping two realities separated and inter-related. Rather, understanding what anything means occurs through our use of language to symbolise meaning in the context of our human culture—further discussed in the next chapter.

John Heaton is critical of Winnicott here. He calls the notion of an inner and outer reality

> a pseudo problem created by misunderstanding our initiation into language. It assumes that the relation between us, other people and the world is an external one rather than being an internal relationship. We cannot get outside ourselves, our language and practices to observe our selves and then wonder how they become related. We are in the world and cannot be separated from it. There can be no "I" or "we" that it makes sense to separate from the world we live in. (2010b, p. 108)

And further:

> The phenomenon of the transitional object occurs as the infant has not developed the concepts of objectivity: the transitional object is neither without nor within; these concepts have no meaning for it. The infant does not have to grow to accept external reality as there is no external reality for it to accept; it is already in the world but has not got the concepts of inner and outer. The transitional object is best understood as part of an early language-game.[26]

---

[26] We can also think of the whole process of using words in the way language functions as one of those games by means of which children learn their native language. I call these games "language-games" (Wittgenstein, 1953, pp. 3–5).

> … There is an internal relation between the acquisition of language and becoming who we are. Our entire linguistic practices imbue our words with life. (2010b, p. 109)

For Heaton, it is not necessary to divide inner from outer any more than it's necessary to divide body from self, or mind from body. Transitional objects, the origins of meaning and the development of a capacity to form meaningful symbols are a way of being in the world and developing an orientation to the world through language.

If a baby needs to rest from anxiety, fear, or worry, say when being left to fall asleep, they rock themselves, sing a little song, suck their thumb, rub a bit of blanket around their upper lip—called transitional phenomena—to soothe, comfort, and relax. Their body agitation settles in relation to being left. I doubt they are relating inner to outer or keeping them separate; rather, they are settling down into a more comfortable relation to what's happening, being left alone, falling asleep. Teddy could be indispensable. Sometimes, nothing works.

When fully awake, the engagement of the child with a transitional object shifts the child's energy, attention, and focus to play while imbuing such play with interest and value. The symbolising function combines speech, thought, imagery, sound, and actual playing in a creative mix and mess of seemingly random noise and movement to those observing it. I call this "embodied symbolisation". It occurs spontaneously for children, if it is not prevented, through play, and through the child's natural engagement with the world. Children are "coming to terms" with the world as they go. They are expressing themselves and crystallising meaning out of their early experiences—Wittgenstein's language games.

There is also a noticeable attempt on the part of babies or small children to incorporate the transitional object into their body or vice versa, to incorporate themselves, the body or parts of it, into the object. Examples are wrapping themselves in a blanket, smothering a teddy, pulling apart a doll, poking a finger into an eye socket, ripping legs off—seeing what is inside, stuffing the corner of cloth into the mouth, grasping the object so tightly—they won't let it go, even when asleep, getting all tangled up in string and so on. Mouthing and sucking tend to be common and practically anything can be taken into the mouth, often to the alarm of parents. All of these activities can be transitional.

The object takes on a special significance to the baby, so special that the teddy bear becomes more important than mother herself, for a time. The child may find it easier to be left alone, for example, with teddy than with any other person.

For adults, when it comes to the endowment of an object with meaning, we have to take responsibility for it or ownership of it rather than insist the meaning is inherent. With insistence, you are open to the attribution that you are operating under an illusion, or worse: suffering from a delusional disorder!

If I say that I love my car (and I do) then you might say, there goes another bloke who loves his car. If I start trying to convince you that my car is the best car in the world, and no one could ever have a car as special as mine and even other people with the same make of car don't have *my* special car—then you may start to think: this bloke is a bit mad (and you would be right).

What if I am forced to sell my car? What if I can only afford a lesser car? Or no car at all?

- Can I feel okay?
- Would I descend into a deep depression?
- Manifest an adjustment disorder?
- Suffer trauma and all the post-traumatic consequences that follow?
- Wallow in self-pity, bemoaning my plight to anyone who will listen?
- Feel humiliated when seen stepping off the bus?
- Would life cease to be worth living?

If your way of symbolising yourself, your concept of yourself, is fixed and cannot allow for changes in life's fortunes, your health, relationships, or, say, ageing, then adverse changes can be devastating, a position commonly encountered by mental health professionals in those who consult them.

In the following chapter, I look at the initiation into language as the means through which symbolisation happens, to gain a deeper understanding of how meaning is formed and expressed.

CHAPTER 5

Language and the body

Understanding meaning cannot be separated from the
fact that we have to be initiated into language.
John M. Heaton

Learning from a two-year-old

Instead of looking into the mind, or studying words, to understand how we make or
fail to make sense, we need to understand the child's initiation into language wherein it
comes to master sense making through the use of signs.

(Heaton, 2010b, pp. 106–107)

I had the good fortune to live for a year with one of my grandchildren from nearly one-and-a-half
to two-and-a-half years old. Over this time, her command of spoken language grew by leaps
and bounds and, in the process, taught me a great deal. The expression "initiation into language" came to life, though every child differs in their way of acquiring language. Out of
respect for her privacy, I will call her Lucy.

From my point of view, the "game" of initiation into language served two primary needs:
(1) for Lucy to express herself and (2) to understand each other. Though there are many other
functions at play, these two were at the forefront. Lucy showed me how language is rooted in
the body. Here are some examples:

- One of her earliest gestures was to raise her shoulders while bending her arms at the elbow
  with palms turned-up, while at the same time her face gestures as if to say "Huh?" Or "What

just happened?" Or "I don't understand that?" Or "That's funny!" So, if we are playing with a ball and it rolls under the dresser before Lucy sees where it goes, while looking for it, she might make this gesture. She is clearly saying "It disappeared! Where did the ball go? I don't see it anywhere" but without words. Hence the use of a sign. The meaning of "language" extends beyond the use of words.

- One of her earliest verbal expressions was "Uh oh". She might say this in different contexts which gave different, but related, meanings. So, a piece of bread falls from her highchair while eating. "Uh oh!"—here this seems to mean, "Oh no, I wanted that and now it has fallen on the floor". But she might also say this playfully, as if pretending to feel loss. Here, she might throw a piece of bread on the floor from her highchair. "Uh oh!" Now, we are playing with loss, deliberately created. Notice how the context changes the meaning of the same expression.

- Crying can have numerous meanings depending on the context and on what is being expressed. There is crying in pain, protest, outrage, for attention, in frustration, anger, sadness, and grief, or even possibly joy—to name a few. It is for you to decipher the difference.

- The full-blown temper tantrum of lying on the floor, screaming, and banging hands and feet is another. To be fair, Lucy never did this. I remember tantrums from raising my own children. The meaning varies—there is a release of pressure, a feral wildness and a defiance expressed as a part of it. It as if the child wants to say "There is nothing you can do to make me stop, to make me feel better or to control me. You are powerless. And I am frustrated to the point of madness!"

- Lucy learned the word "no" early on. However, "no" could be said in many different ways, with different inflexions in her tone of voice, and different hand gestures and overall body movements as to give quite a different sense. There was the simple "no" that just meant no. There was the annoyed "no" that said "I really do not want to do that". There was the defiant "no" that means "I am the boss, and I will decide". There was the agreeable "no" as in "Do you want any more dinner, Lucy? No, finished now". And there was the combative "no" that indicates "I will fight you to get my way". And so on.

- "Yes" came a bit later and was harder to say. "Yeth, yesh, yeh"; there were also many variations of meaning depending on how it was said.

- Hitting and kicking, not so much Lucy's thing—but other kids hit and kick as a means of expression through their bodies' contact with yours. Recently, I was kicked by a not-quite two-year-old; it strangely felt like a combination of aggression and affection. Her cheeky grin suggested she was playing with me but was the game one of aggression or affection? Or both?

- Pointing. Not all children point, and some do more than others. From an early age Lucy would point with clear intention to what she wanted to have or know about or bring our attention to. The pointing was specific. She liked ceiling fans, and if one was off, pointing to it meant turn it on. She liked the iPad and pointing meant she wanted to play a game.

She liked bananas and avocados, dolls and stuffed animals and she liked to play ball with me, knowing I like playing ball. In most cases, pointing said "I want that".[27]

In these examples, the body is used to express and communicate, to convey meaning. You cannot look up in a dictionary what shrugging shoulders means, or pointing, or crying. Conversely, you *can* look up every word there is, but you won't necessarily discover what anyone means by their use of that word. Socialisation and, specifically, social communication, begins with gestures.

> "The spoken word is a gesture, and its meaning, a world."
> (Merleau-Ponty, 1962, p. 184)

Meaning is intentional, not referential

Meaning is both personal and interpersonal, it is determined by context, history, and the culture in which it is expressed. Meaning depends upon relationship and varies from one relationship to the next. And meaning varies at different points in time. To understand anyone, you need to gain a sense of how their body moves in their way of speaking and gesturing. A very young baby will appear disturbed if they smile at their primary caregiver and that person doesn't respond in kind, or more so if that person doesn't respond at all.[28] So, if mother is preoccupied or distracted by her mobile phone, or watching TV, and turns away from her baby's beseeching contact, baby will show something: anxiety, distress, concern, dismay, protest, or sorrow. This is well before words appear on the scene. Babies within a week or two weeks old can differentiate between the language of their primary carers and a foreign language (Heaton, 2010a, p. 131). This is because babies are already exposed to the language of their mothers in the womb and so can differentiate the sounds of another language by the time they are born (Ramirez, 2016).

The same principles—meaning depends upon context and relationship—apply when words do appear on the scene. Doctors and mental health professionals can get into difficulties when

---

[27] In child development, there are two types of pointing: (1) protoimperative is desire for an object and (2) protodeclarative is to direct attention and share experience. Usually, protoimperative comes first, then protodeclarative. Lack of pointing can be a flag for a possible Autistic Spectrum Disorder.

[28] This comes from the Developmental Psychologist Ed Tronick and what is called "the still-face paradigm"—a study highlighting the toddler's ability to cope with maternal unavailability. It supported the idea that children in their first year of life are attempting to make meaning out of an event like a mother with a still-face (no expression or responsiveness) against their expectations.

they understand language as referential. That means that the words a patient uses means something that is pre-determined and can be translated or interpreted according to a pre-existing lexicon (like a dictionary or the DSM, but also like scientific language or psychoanalytic theory). An example of this occurs in this clinical vignette:

A patient complained of a frog in her throat. She couldn't speak properly because of this. Her voice was raspy and constricted. Sometimes, she couldn't speak at all because she choked on her words and couldn't get them out. She believed there was something *in* there obstructing her vocal cords.

She went to her doctor who examined her and could see nothing there. He sent her for further tests that produced no explanation of her speech disorder. She was so insistent that there was something *in* her throat, the doctor referred her to a psychologist.

She had one session with a psychologist and was told she was mistaken and needed to correct an error in her thinking. Later, she told me she found this invalidating—"she didn't take me seriously"—and so never went back. (Even if cognitive behavioural therapy had convinced her to think differently, there would be no understanding of what it meant.) She went back to her GP who then referred her to a psychiatrist.

To the psychiatrist, her insistence that there was something physical in her throat, despite evidence to the contrary, meant it was obvious she had a delusional disorder. After a token history-taking, the diagnosis was made, and medications prescribed. Indeed, her literal thinking led the psychiatrist to suspect she had a psychotic condition and to prescribe anti-psychotic medications. Instead of helping her feel better or making her speech easier, it made her feel foggy-headed, sleepy, and unfocused, and it became even harder to speak. Then, she felt like a zombie with a frog in her throat, she later told me.

She consulted me seeking a different approach, her fourth attempt. I listened to her description of her difficulties and asked about its onset (the *When-did-you-first-notice-these-symptoms?* question is Therapy 101). She said that the frog appeared in her throat two months ago following a critical attack by her husband when she complained that he had been "shutting her down". She felt every time she disagreed with him or expressed a different opinion he flew into a rage and shouted at her. This time was the worst.

I said: "So you developed a condition that prevents you from speaking, from expressing yourself in a way that gets you into trouble with your husband."

She seemed surprised at the connection but agreed it made sense. She looked upset and concerned at this and when I inquired as to what she was feeling, she said: "But I was sure there was actually an obstruction there and I couldn't understand why the doctor couldn't see it. To tell you the truth, I would rather have a medical condition than blame Jean-Pierre. He gets so mad at me."

I said: "I don't see it as a question of blame but rather how you are affected by your husband." I paused, thinking about it. Then I continued: "Jean-Pierre—your husband is

French? And you're English. Isn't "frog" the derogatory nickname the English call the French?"

There was no need for further appointments because her voice cleared *miraculously*.

Notice how this patient thought there was something inside her. The doctor also thought there might be something inside her such as a bacterial infection but couldn't find anything. Then, the psychiatrist thought there was something inside her (mind), a delusion about an obstruction—an example of "the disease of the mind" approach. I sought first to put in context her issue and make a connection with her primary relationship. Secondly, I had a conversation with her about what was *expressed* by her condition and her way of *symbolising* it, that is, her way of representing it. In other words, what is the function of not speaking? What does it mean? Of what use is it? The expression "frog-in-your-throat" usually means speaking with a croaky voice (like a frog). The important thing here was not to diagnose her based on a symptom of a mental disorder, rather to *understand* what was being expressed through her physical condition (pre-symbolically) and her manner of speaking about it. Her use of language is her way of symbolising.

In considering what something means,
don't assume it doesn't exist.

What it means shows why it exists. Of course, believing there is an actual frog in your throat when there isn't *is* a delusion. The psychiatrist isn't wrong, but the approach isn't helpful. Nothing *therapeutic* is understood by calling it a delusion and, in this case, medication compounds the issue rather than helps. If anything, like so many patients, this one felt frustrated by not being believed, and invalidated by the assumption there was something wrong with her. To say *her belief is delusional* is a proposition that exists in a cultural context and represents a particular type of perspective. It is a way of seeing this patient's condition. It's not the only way and not necessarily the best, even if it is true. It might be the least therapeutic in the sense of healing the soul.

What's missed in these mental and physical health practices and what is also often missed in considering the bigger questions of meaning and what makes life worth living is attention to symbolisation. Symbolisation refers to the use of language to express meaning. In the example above, the patient's difficulty speaking was symbolised as "there is a frog in my throat".

A woman believes she has an actual frog in her throat. The doctor, psychologist, and psychiatrist all understand her to have a delusion, as no actual frog can be found in her throat. They are not wrong, but they have also not understood her, or, specifically what she means when she says this. Their frame of reference is objectivity, and as such it is referential. *Is there a frog or isn't there?* Objectively, there is no frog—therefore thinking there is one is irrational. This patient is wrong and needs to be convinced of it. They are right, but their approach doesn't work. It is oppositional. They have missed this patient's intention in her manner of speaking, and so they have missed her meaning.

The way you use language is intentional, personal, and temporal. It occurs at a set point of time. To understand language as referential is to render it atemporal and generalised. For mental health practices, if we understand patients through their referential meanings, what is understood becomes abstracted from its context, and as such, depersonalised. This process easily becomes a source of confusion and argument. The meaning is debatable. The depersonalisation of meaning debases mental health and is, therefore, counter-therapeutic.

Meanwhile, the patient can hardly speak because of this "frog". Not being understood makes it worse and being *medicated* makes it worse again. As so often the case, this patient now has a condition compounded by diagnoses and treatments.

Referential meanings can be found in reference books such as dictionaries, *Gray's Anatomy*, or psychiatric textbooks. The patient's meaning is not determined by finding the right reference book in which to look it up. Again, you won't find what this patient means in the DSM or International Classification of Diseases (ICD) by classifying the patterns of patients' symptoms or mental disorders into pathological syndromes. (That is the bigger delusion!)

> To understand anyone, learn what they *mean*.

The meaning of the expression "frog in her throat" is found in her body, in the way it functions, in preventing her from speaking easily. The word "frog" could be interpreted as a derogatory colloquialism for her French husband; also useful is its function of helping her stay out of trouble with him. She is punished for voicing opinions that differ from his. Part of the confusion is seeking help from a medical practitioner who will look for organic causes, or from a psychologist who will attempt to change the way she thinks about this, or from a psychiatrist who diagnoses a mental disorder requiring medication. I see these sorts of confusions regularly in my practice in less extreme examples. It can be difficult to know who to consult about what.

In this example, the experience of a frog in her throat that prevents her from speaking is a pre-symbolic expression because the patient herself does not know what it means. It is a psychosomatic symptom because her body is expressing a personal meaning without words. The body *speaks* in pre-symbolic ways. Not speaking in words says something. The aim of therapy is to convert the pre-symbolic meanings into an intentional use of language so that they can become part of a conversation. Meaningful conversations promote understanding and thereby open possibilities for change and relief of suffering.

What occurs in her body is not a frog but rather a difficulty speaking that she conceptualises, indeed believes, is caused by a literal frog obstructing her speech. She is surprised the doctor cannot find it, much less remove it. It is disembodied even though it occurs in and affects her body because it is split off from what the condition means. To convert a disembodied pre-symbolic form of expression into one that is embodied and symbolised requires formulating in words the meaning of the experience. It takes a dead metaphor and brings it to life. Its meaning is not simply a product of an intellectual or scientific analysis. The term "embodied symbolisation" refers to felt experience expressed in language to another in the context of a relationship where it matters. If the relationship is with a mental health professional, it becomes more important that it matters. If it doesn't matter, whatever treatment or therapy is given is less likely to be effective. This can even apply to medications because the psychology underlying their effectiveness is both personal and interpersonal. People do not necessarily respond to medications in the same way. Bodies are not identical. And the relationship with the prescribing professional can make a difference to the efficacy of the medication (Krupnick et al., 1996, p. 537). The way a person is embodied—its uniqueness—is brought to the interpersonal interface of a professional relationship.

Embodied symbolisation means that what is expressed is meaningful. Indeed, it is the embodiment of symbolisation that *makes it* meaning-full in the context of mattering to someone else.

> Understanding the meaning of embodied symbolisation involves listening through an attitude of not-knowing.[29]

Dis/embodied

In the example of Clarissa (Chapter 3), her sexual experience is disembodied because she *had to* be drunk to be sexual which, in turn, prevented her from feeling as much in her body as she would have otherwise and for her partner. If not for the volume of alcohol, she would have been able to remember it. She cannot afford embodied symbolisation because it would mean too much to her. She would merge with her lover, and she knows this would get her into all kinds of hot water, and has in the past, especially with her very first deep love, Adrian, who exited her life traumatically by exiting his. With her current partner, Paul, she already feels

---

[29] This is the opposite of the medical model, used by psychology, that strives for expertise. Paradoxically, professional expertise can be counter-therapeutic, and conversely therapists may know a great deal but are most effective when they disavow expertise. (Every bit of psychoeducation can be Googled.) A therapist needs to know the client afresh each session.

that she wants this relationship to mean *everything*, though with past partners, sex has meant absolutely nothing.

In Chapter 3, I also referenced R. D. Laing who described the split between body and self—dis/embodiment—as an attempt to create safety and protect the self from the threat of disintegration, a consequence of unbearable pain. With Paul, the slightest hint of withdrawal—not responding to a text message straightaway—is like a knife in the heart for Clarissa. She struggles to cope with it.

His choice of words makes a world of difference. If he says "I need to go away for a weekend to get some space"—the "I" indicates separateness which creates emotional pain for Clarissa. Similarly, if he says "I'm going to see a band" instead of "Let's go see a band" or "Would you like to go with me to see a band?" or "We could go see this band I want to hear"—the former is the expression of a separate, individual person (of course, she could say "I'd like to hear that band, too" but Clarissa is sensitised to what Paul wants)—instead of the latter in which it is implicit they will go together. The difference is a world of pain or a world of joy.

Symbolisation refers to putting into words what you want to say. Words can be hollow and empty just as a person can feel hollow and empty. Feeling like that will make it easy for the words used to feel like they don't mean much. As I said in *How Two Love* (Resnick, 2016), say what you mean and mean what you say. That is a good start in the move towards embodied symbolisation within the context of a relationship. Though it is perfectly possible to make a general statement whole-heartedly such as "I love my car", or "I hate politicians", or "I wish the sun would come out", or "I would like to kill my internet service provider"—who you are saying this to and your reasons for saying it make a difference to its meaning and degree of embodiment.

In embodied symbolisation, language is not restricted only to words. So much meaning is also conveyed unspoken (see Stern, 2019). The domain of language goes way beyond the spoken word. Everything about the way you look, move, speak, write, and act can be understood as linguistic. Gesticulations are part of language; they are as expressive as words, if not more so. Indeed, it would be hard to understand what anyone's gestures mean if not understood linguistically. If I pick up the bare handle of a frying pan from the stove not realising it had just been exposed to a high flame, then "OWWWWW!" expresses the pain of pure burning sensation. That is still a linguistic expression. Even if no sound came out of my mouth at all, and I grimaced silently in pain—this is also a linguistic expression. If someone is there, I would say it is a communication. If no one is there, it is still expressive. What is being expressed here is only an experience of pure physical sensation, yet remains of the linguistic order.

A transcendent experience, a spiritual experience, an experience of deep meditation, and an experience of at-one-ment with the world, or God, or The Cosmos is more than likely going to happen in total silence. No words can express the ineffable. Words struggle to express the ethereal. Yet, these experiences are still linguistic because once we have acquired language, experience is, itself, a function of language as language is a function of experience. You could not conceptualise your experience as sacred, or transcendent, or spiritual without language even if there are no words to say what that experience is. Some thinkers have identified God as that which cannot be conceptualised (though this is tangential). Accordingly, God is that which no human mind can define, though many have tried, and some insist on their definition, or murder other people if you don't agree—in the name of God. Dogmatism is not divinity.

> As God is not an object, God cannot be known objectively.

Whether by God or a force of nature, you are given the possibility of a full sense of embodiment. But disembodiment seems more the norm than the exception.

More of what I learned from Lucy

Returning to the acquisition of language, when I think of my experience of Lucy learning language for the first time, some observations emerge:

1) She is being constantly bathed in language, she is swimming in it, she is immersed in it, it washes over her as she goes.
2) Her orientation to the world, to human activity, and to other people, is being formed by her immersion in language, specifically the very human speech that occurs all around her, to her and in relation to her (this corresponds with the formation of a self).
3) When she speaks or gestures or communicates, there is an intention being expressed. There is a logic in her intention, it may be her own "internal" logic but the key to understanding her intention is to understand her personal logic. Personal logic is what psycho-logical means, in my use of it.
4) The logic of intention is contextual. The context in which her meaning emerges is essential to its sense. Extrapolating from there, understanding practically anyone, practically any time, requires an understanding of the context in which they are communicating their personal logic of intention.[30]
5) Part of the context is your relation to another person. Meaning depends on relationship, and relationship is the well-spring of the context of meaning. Even writing this sentence only makes sense because of the writer's idea of his reader. Is this a relationship? No, but yes. It is a potential or imaginary relationship. The structure of relationship is contained there as a source of context—when I write, I am speaking to someone, an other, though I don't know "you" and so "you" are my imaginary object, or more accurately, a concept. I have a fantasy of readers hungrily devouring my words.

---

[30] This is one problem with text messages; it can be impossible to know their context. And why they are rife with misunderstandings. Text needs context.

6) Another part of context is history. History gives meaning to culture, it puts flesh on the bones, and both give meaning to the logic of intention. Who you are and the position you occupy are constituted by your history and the history of your culture. This is easier to see in a small child.

7) There is no language without the body. Language bodies forth. Language is an action of the body. And speech, writing, communication, and all forms of expressiveness are activities of the body, require a body, and, typically, derive their greatest weight through their embodiment.

8) Meaning-fullness occurs when the above are all happening in sync, a harmonious equilibrium of human relatedness. This is facilitated by attunement to the other person, empathy, compassion, thought, care, and love.

Understanding the observations above serve as a good basis for any mental health practice.

Connectedness, both personal and professional, makes your use of language meaningful, and meaningfulness makes your life worth living.

> As a child, childhood is your greatest teacher.
> As an adult, children are your greatest teachers.
> As a senior, a baby is your greatest teacher.

For me, one of the great miracles of early development is the learning of language and the rainbow diversity of children's expressiveness. You could say a word to Lucy, and she would repeat it though never having heard it before. "Galah", "taxi", "fish tank", "spaghetti", "polar bear", and "Jimi Hendrix". But when it came to "broccoli"—a pretty hard word—she could say it, but it often sounded like "brockabi". Part of the miracle of language acquisition is the miracle of memory.

My other granddaughter, not quite two years old, has taken to calling herself "Honey Bee". Recently, she saw a statue of the Buddha in my garden. She pointed and was told "that is the Buddha". Three or four weeks later, she saw a small sculpture at her other grandparent's home and said "Buddha". Her granny couldn't believe she knew that word and had remembered the name having only heard it only once.

Me: What do you want for lunch?
Lucy: Brockabi.

"Brockabi" is a word-sign, it symbolises "broccoli". What difference does it make if she asks for brockabi or broccoli? I know exactly what she means, what she intends, what she wants, equally. The important thing is to understand what people mean by the signs they use to symbolise. This is important in every relationship and crucial in the consulting room of a mental health professional.

Thank you to Lucy and Honey Bee.

Patients use words mistakenly all the time. My role as a therapist is not to correct them, not to find some hidden meaning deep in the unconscious to theorise the meaning of the mistake, but rather to understand what they mean by their use or misuse of words. It will only matter for Lucy and Honey Bee when they go to school and have to use words correctly.

Speaking truthfully

John Heaton writes about a therapy patient who insisted her therapist was keeping her thoughts in a drawer of his desk. This accusation was repeated angrily for months on end. We need to understand this patient's own internal logic to make sense out of this statement which on the face of it, makes no sense.

> Logic is not a set of general laws which rule sense. (Heaton, 2010b, p. 113)

Psychiatry, psychology, and some psychoanalysis and psychotherapy practices can make the mistake of trying to assess whether a proposition is objectively true or not. If you regard the patient's statement above as false—because it cannot be true, as thoughts cannot be kept in drawers, other than in the form of written notes (but that is not what she meant)—then you would be correct. And yet, this patient was speaking truthfully. She was speaking truthfully without speaking the truth because these are two quite distinct and separate positions.

Understanding language as referential, based on what words refer to in a general way, brings confusion to logic in realms of human experience and, especially, mental suffering. Many try to "correct" what patients think or say as if professionals already know what is right, true, and correct. Understanding personal meaning is not and cannot be an empirical science.[31] It can be a science (remember: from the Latin *scire* to know) in the heuristic and hermeneutic sense, in the sense of knowing what someone means through discovery and interpretation. Consider the patient in the example above:

---

[31] This is the mistake of many contemporary academic psychologists. "Correcting errors in your thinking" indicates the psychologist must know what you should mean, the truth, the rational, what is correct, at the outset. As an example of this, during a recent supervision session, a developmental paediatrician was distressed by a heated argument with a psychologist over whether a child should be diagnosed as autistic. The psychologist was one hundred per cent certain this child was autistic and couldn't fathom why the paediatrician was unwilling to diagnose accordingly. They argued at length. Finally, the paediatrician asked: "Have you ever seen this child?" The psychologist answered: "No, I have only seen the child's mother."

Briefly, her mother was a professional expert on how to bring up children. She had fixed rules throughout the day as to how children ought to behave. Everything, including play, was elaborately planned by her. The patient grew up not recognising that she had a mind of her own.

Given this upbringing, it made sense that this woman accused the therapist of keeping her mind in a drawer. She had no concept of the possibility of a meeting of minds without one trying to obliterate the other. It was important that the therapist respected the woman's fixed belief and did not, like her mother, try and impose "reality" on it. The woman was speaking truthfully when she had the courage to insist that her mind was in the therapist's drawer. To explain it as a delusion, a false belief, is to confuse truth with speaking truthfully. This leads to treating her brain chemically or her mind psychoanalytically, or her thoughts by cognitive techniques; this also assumes there is a real meaning which the experts know. These would be another way of obliterating her mind. It was only by allowing her language to show what she said that she was enabled to enjoy a meeting of minds with her therapist.

… Meaning is not an act of an individual mind or mental picture. Neither is logic a set of rules that must be applied to language nor is logical syntax concerned with the proscription of combinations of signs or symbols. Rather, it enables the signs we use, when we give voice to our thoughts and feelings, to symbolise. (Heaton, 2010b, p. 114)

Symbolisation

I use the term "symbolisation" as a coming-to-terms in a double sense. First, coming to terms means formulating in words, and second it means coming to terms with the way it is. The expression "coming to terms" means accepting something for what it is, even if it is not what you want or not what you thought.

> Realise that things are not what you thought must be,
> or that things are what you thought could not be.

The patient described above is again an example of disembodiment, expressed graphically in the proposition that the therapist has her thoughts or mind in a drawer. Embodiment requires ownership of your own mind, your own thoughts, and feelings—embodied—as a part of you. Mind is not to be confused with brain, even if a healthy mind requires a functioning brain. Embodiment does not mean your brain lives in your skull. It means your thoughts and feelings are your own, even if they cannot be located in any particular place in your body. Thoughts may feel as if they happen in the head. Feelings may feel as if they happen in the pit of your stomach, or back of your throat or centre of your heart. Perceptions may feel they happen in your eyes, nose, mouth, ears, or fingertips. However, embodied symbolisation refers to an integration of your being in the context of your orientation to the world, and your relationships with other people. How you communicate, how you express yourself, how you reach others and are reached by them is the heart and soul of who you are and what things mean to you.

Meaning emerges in the ways we affect each other. Some days, I wake feeling rough; not always, but that happens. I go to my office and sit down with my first patient. Immediately, how I feel changes. The former roughness is smoothed out. I want to know about this person. When I say "How are you?" I want to know. I care. Any therapist that doesn't should do something else. I mean it. Even when the reply comes back "Same shit, different day", I remain attentive. That is the job. Then we go into it. I am taken out of myself. The rough feeling has vanished. Sometimes I think to myself "Seeing patients makes me feel better, I really hope seeing me does something for them". It is very noticeable. When the next person comes in, I feel different again. I am affected. It's the same, but different. It means something. This person's mood or mental state is different from that of the previous person, and so on. I take note of how I'm affected. I don't know exactly what it means. Yet. I want to find out. I notice my bodily being is affected. I feel anxious with one person, excited with another, tense with a third, and a warm feeling of anticipation for another. I'm affected by this next one before that person even arrives, just the thought of them. Sometimes, there is dread.

Some people's suffering is dreadful. And frankly, some people are dreadful. I'm not the only one who feels that. The good news is: if you work at it, and therapy works—the dreadful person becomes less so and may well grow to be more agreeable or even delightful company. Even better if others experience this change in the same way. Part of the process may be to come to terms with your dreadfulness, or to put it in a milder way, what other people find disagreeable.

Coming to terms means finding words and sometimes accepting that which you most do not want to be the case.

There is a third sense of "coming to terms" in the context of a commercial deal. You reach mutually agreeable terms for an exchange to proceed. This has relevance, too—sometimes a negotiation with "the ways things are" is necessary for movement to happen, almost like a business contract. Not only commercially, sometimes we come to terms with each other for our relationships to work, to negotiate with each other successfully.

Therapists are learners, not experts

In therapy, it works best to practice with your L-plates on (the Australian learner's permit for driving). I've been at it a long time now. Some people see me as a professional expert. But the nature of the work reflects the indeterminate nature of each patient's individual experience. I joke that I've been practicing for forty-something years and I'm beginning to get the hang of it. Actually, it's true. I don't know how anyone will be until they come in and tell me—even with patients I have seen for some time. Here is a further example from my earlier work with Clarissa:

Clarissa came in and told me she had had a mental breakdown a few days previously. "From the moment I woke up to the moment I went to sleep, all I could think about was where do I stand with Paul. Everyone thinks I'm completely chill. That is what I show them. When asked, I say everything is great. But inside I feel completely crazy. I was so distressed I couldn't go to work, I stayed home and cried literally the whole day. Paul doesn't know I feel this way. He's gone away for a couple of weeks. He needed some space. I understand that. When I think of him, I realise how much he has going on and it makes sense. He isn't saying he needs space from me, just all the pressure he's under. I get it. Logically. But my feelings are so irrational. I keep rehearsing a speech to break up with him. I can't be with him. It's not enough. I need someone who doesn't disappear, who stays in touch with me and answers my texts without four hours going by. With me it's all or nothing. If it's not *all*, I can't do it. Now I feel completely empty again."

Clarissa was broken-down, crying, and distressed while telling me this. Most of the session was spent with her sobbing. I felt concerned, I could feel her distress. It was palpable. It was painful. She was tormented. It was hard to know what to say. For all my supposed expertise, I could only try to contain her, be present, emotionally attuned, and empathic: what Winnicott called "a holding environment". Mostly, I just listened and stayed connected through her emotional outpouring, tears, mucous, and pain. She left determined to break up her relationship—a relationship that seemed better for her than most, if not all, of her previous ones—and I feared that would make her feel worse.

I thought about her over the course of the next week. When she came back for her next appointment, she looked better, happier. I noticed this as I passed through the waiting area to my room after lunch and glanced at her playing with her phone. I noticed a feeling of relief wash over me, I relaxed physically, felt receptive and easier about the session to come. When she came in, she told me she felt instantly better after the last session (I had no idea). I blurted out what I had been containing since the previous session as it isn't right to say it when someone is so distressed (there is expertise in knowing when to keep your mouth shut!).

"All I really needed to do was to fuckn cry", she said. I said that I had thought of her and about our last session and then I continued: "I would ask you to consider giving up this all-or-nothing position. Give it up, if you can. I think it is key to much of your suffering. You can't have *all*. The only time anyone gets 'all' is when they are a newborn baby and that is if they're lucky enough to have a primary carer who is highly responsive to their dependency needs. If you hold out for 'all' you wind up with nothing and feel empty. Paul is into you; he didn't leave to get away from you. He just needed space, something you understood. It's a good relationship and it would be a shame to end it, especially when nothing has happened between you to be cause for leaving."

Clarissa's response was interesting, and unexpected (good thing for L-plates). "Yes, I have been thinking along similar lines. And I felt so much better after last session, I was able to think about it more rationally. I will stay in it for now and see where it goes with Paul. But he is only eight months out of a long marriage, he is preoccupied with an acrimonious settlement process, he has debts that are worrying him, he plays in a band that has its own issues and he is stressed at work. It's true that he is really into me, and it's true that we work well when we're together. But I don't think he is really ready for a full relationship. And I am ready. I want to love someone right now, and someone who can love me back just as fully. The other issue is that I definitely do not want children. One hundred per cent—this is not negotiable. We have never had this discussion, but he is thirty-nine and doesn't have any and I could imagine that is something he will want. So, I'm not sure this is going to work long-term in any case."

I was struck by how clear, balanced, mature, and logical her thinking about all this was. Opposite to the week before, Clarissa was no longer overcome by emotion, so she could think logically and meaningfully about where she stood in relation to Paul (not just the other way around) and where he stood in his own life. It felt embodied, as she said it. There was nothing of the previous sense of fusion or merging. She could be a separate person.

If I was a professional expert who knew in advance what she needed to change into, she would not have arrived at her own position, of her own accord, in her own time. There is a different sense of expertise involved in recognising this.

This is an example of embodied symbolisation. Clarissa needed to "fuckn cry"[32]—she needed to ground her feelings in her body. True she felt overtaken by her emotions but expressed in the context of our working relationship and therapeutic process, the meaning of her emotions moves her in the direction of integration. She comes together in herself. Feels better. And from there she can come to terms with how she sees her relationship with Paul, what she wants, how it affects her, the potential problems and issues ahead and the implications for the future. It is not all. It is not nothing. It is what it is.

Her way of expressing her reflections[33] is crystal clear, feels real, is grounded in her own personal truth, and so is embodied. It belongs to her whole being as a person and is integrated within herself and then between us as she expresses it. She has come to terms with it.

We can work with that.

---

[32] The word "fuckn" is important here. If you recall Chapter 3, Clarissa had severe judgements that she held against herself for how she felt, and I take this word to be an echo of her contempt for herself based on feelings like this one: the need to cry. She could have said: "I just needed to cry."

[33] This is a good example of what Peter Fonagy and his researchers (Fonagy, Gergely, Jurist, & Target, 2004) call "affective mentalization" (more on this later).

Contemporary perspectives on trauma, the body, and language

Trauma, uncontrollable emotions, bodily symptoms, and the place of language and its relation to embodiment lead me to look at some of the contemporary literature on these issues. Bessel van der Kolk writes:

> Almost every brain-imaging study of trauma patients finds abnormal activation of the insula. This part of the brain integrates and interprets the input from the internal organs—including our muscles, joints, and balance (proprioceptive) system—to generate the sense of being embodied. The insula can transmit signals to the amygdala that trigger fight/flight responses. This does not require any cognitive input or any conscious recognition that something has gone awry—you just feel on edge and unable to focus or, at worst, have a sense of imminent doom. These powerful feelings are generated deep inside the brain and cannot be eliminated by reason or understanding.
>
> … Only by getting in touch with your body, by connecting viscerally with your self, can you regain a sense of who you are, your priorities and values … In order to overcome trauma, you need help to get back in touch with *your body,* with *your Self.*
>
> There is no question that language is essential: Our sense of Self depends on being able to organize our memories into a coherent whole. (2104, p. 247, original emphasis)

Van der Kolk's book shows how traumatic experience is stored in the body; it is useful for therapists and patients alike. Although he says powerful feelings cannot be eliminated by reason or understanding, I don't think we (therapists) are setting out to eliminate anyone's feelings. As I see it, when we speak of connecting viscerally, or regaining a sense of who you are, or getting in touch with your body—this is the role of embodied symbolisation, as I see it. What kind of *sense* of who you are could you make without reason or understanding? To me, this sense of sense doesn't make sense.

Pat Ogden and colleagues argue that we need to differentiate and integrate top-down and bottom-up therapeutic approaches. Top-down means starting with cognition (head) and working to emotions (feelings) and then to the body whereas bottom-up is the reverse. This is how she puts it:

> Top-down cortically mediated techniques typically use cognition to regulate affect and sensorimotor experience, focusing on meaning making and understanding. The entry point is the story, and the formulation of a coherent narrative is of prime importance. A linguistic sense of self is fostered in this process, and experience changes through understanding.[34] In bottom-up approaches, the body's sensation and movement are the entry points, and changes in sensorimotor experience are used to support self-regulation,

---

[34] Notice this is the opposite of what van der Kolk said above.

memory processing, and success in daily life. Meaning and understanding emerge from new experiences rather than the other way around. Through bottom-up interventions, a shift in the somatic sense of self in turn affects the linguistic sense of self. Sensorimotor psychotherapy blends these bottom-up interventions, which directly address movement, sensory experience, and body sensation, with top-down approaches and verbal dialogue. (Ogden, Minton, & Pain, 2006, p. 166)

Top-down approaches are often referred to as traditional talking therapies and bottom-up approaches as sensorimotor or trauma-informed therapies. In my own work, I have always done both and have not been aware of there being two different approaches that need blending. The distinction between the two approaches seems somewhat artificial to me but maybe some do only one and some do only the other. The emphasis on the body, on bodily feelings and sensations, on self-awareness and mindfulness of the present moment experience is all important in working with patients trying to heal and recover from trauma, especially early and complex trauma—it is important for everyone.

What is a somatic sense of self if not a semantic sense of self? What kind of sense can you have without language; it doesn't make sense. We have sensations that words cannot express. As soon as we speak about a *sense* of self, then language is invoked. Even a somatic sense of self must depend on concepts that refer to physical experience. If I, as a therapist draw your attention to how your body is feeling or appears, or if I direct you to move in a particular way and ask you what you feel, you will need language to convey a description of your experience. Is that expressing your semantic sense of self or your somatic self? Or both? Does it make sense to separate these two? Isn't this separation the very thing that needs to be overcome?[35]

> If theory divides up experience
> how will therapy restore wholeness?

The stress and distress of post-traumatic experience is the very consequence of disembodiment and the corresponding inability to express oneself in language. Such experience splits a somatic self from a semantic self. As is well documented in the trauma literature, this affects everything. Dissociation occurs as a consequence of the split between language and the body. Dissociation is a form of disembodiment and hence the inability to symbolise (put the meaning of your experience into words, coming to terms with it). It is critical in working with trauma and its consequences not to split off the body, as a "thing"-in-itself. If we abstract the body in thought, we cannot hope to affect integration in practice.

---

[35] This undergirds my thinking of embodied symbolisation.

Following Antonio Damasio, Ogden claims:

> The sense of self is first and foremost a bodily sense, experienced not through language but through sensations and movements of the body. (Ogden, Minton, & Pain, 2006, p. 42)

I don't know what a bodily sense of self could possibly mean if not understood through language. Remember the burning handle of the pan on the stove? "%#&$@! OOWWW!!"—this is pure sensation. It doesn't have meaning until conceptualised in language: "that fucking hurt!" now can become part of my sense of self. A sense of self is historical, contextual, and relational. *Who* you are depends on how you are situated in your world with respect to the meaning of your experience. If I sit in the lotus position in silent meditation, and you say "Bring your attention to your body, start with your toes, and work your way up, notice how you feel"—you are directing me to get in touch with my bodily sense of self. Meanwhile, my thoughts are articulating this experience "My foot is starting to cramp, that pain in my left hip is escalating, my breathing is a little shallow, and my neck feels stiff". What could awareness of your bodily experience possibly mean without language? I burnt my hand on that frying pan! That is a post-symbolic semantic expression of the earlier experience of my bodily sense of self, the physical sensation of "OOWWW!"

As Lucy showed me at the earliest age and stage, her sense of self resided in the unfolding interplay between her body, her developing grasp of language, the physical world, and her significant others that populate it.

Ogden and her colleagues focus on the nervous system and on regulating arousal in the post-traumatic condition. If we abstract the body from the person, we have disconnected, divorced, and even dissociated the person from themselves and also from us. This is the very consequence of trauma that we are trying to overcome by the therapeutic methods informed by such dissociation. Dissociation is, in one way of looking at it, a void of the possible meanings of your experience. The abstraction of *the body* as a concept that is then removed from the person whose body it is—as if you could even entertain a concept without language to conceive it—is, itself, a post-traumatic condition that generates and perpetuates such a void. Perhaps we are all already so traumatised that we fail to see a person as a person but rather as a body that is misfiring or an arousal mechanism that requires regulating? The emperor, indeed, has no clothes. (This is why I turn to Lucy as my teacher.)

You can have physical feelings or sensations without words. You can have nonverbal experience. If we are speaking about a trauma-informed therapy that aims to overcome dissociation, then the meaning of those feelings or sensations will require concepts expressed through language in the service of integration. What needs to be integrated?—what is felt with what it means, where it comes from, processing the past to move on into the present, overcoming the disconnections between them.

There has been an explosion of literature on trauma and how to work with survivors in therapy. The emphasis on the body is right. Perhaps the traditional talking therapies have not focused enough on bodily considerations. And adjunct practices like yoga (especially), massage, acupuncture, EFT, dance, and movement, breathwork, etc., have a role. EMDR has been impressive for trauma, though not without notable exceptions. And sensorimotor psychotherapy has value. Many therapists, myself included, have used Dan Siegel's idea of the "window of tolerance" (1999, p. 341) to good effect, clinically. All mental health practices need to be trauma-informed. In the process, however, separating "the body" out as a thing-in-itself is as much of a mistake as overlooking it completely.

Language, and its central place, in working with trauma, does not have to be limited to the use of words. Music, art, and dance are examples of a kind of language that does not rely upon a verbal idiom. The images of dreams, the grunt and groan of an elderly person getting up out of a chair, the frown of an unhappy child, being waved on by a traffic cop, photos on social media, and the clapping of hands to scare away the crows are all examples of nonverbal language. You don't have to have words to say something meaningful. To arrive at an understanding of meaning, words help to reflect, consider, contemplate, interpret, and then communicate. Communication without words is happening all the time but words are useful if we are to have a conversation about the meaning of it and arrive at a mutual understanding.

Contemporary writing on trauma and on relational psychoanalysis and psychotherapy emphasises that change comes from new experiences. If you think about it, every experience is a new experience. That is all there is: new experiences. You have been there and done that. You have experienced this, countless times before. Same old. It isn't. Even if you have the *same* experience over and again, you have never-before had it this time. That is what mindfulness is about. This is key to living—the recognition of the freshness of the present moment; it is what makes new experience new. What this means in practice is to re-fresh yourself to your own unfolding experience, as it happens. This is precisely what trauma makes so difficult and what needs to be overcome; the struggle to be present in the present.

Reflection on the obstacles to being present furthers the process of therapeutic change, recovery from trauma, and development generally. Working with the body helps but doesn't preclude the need for reflection. Noticing that your inner narrative is different, has shifted ground from its customary pattern, is desirable, and a function of reflection. A new generative understanding that occurs spontaneously from moving or holding your body differently or an insight gleaned from your personal history—both involve reflection. Reflection makes sense in the present of what has occurred without words in the past. This is what makes developmental psychotherapy developmental.

For Donnel B. Stern, there is also something that happens before reflection is possible, regarding what he calls "unformulated experience". He says: "explicit reflection does not constitute the only means by which therapeutic action is accomplished". He believes that nonverbal events are also "primary in the creation of therapeutic action" (2019, p. 16). The professional relationship offers something new and different from past experience. In time, new understandings evolve as the sedimented patterns of experience are disrupted and, to some degree, dismantled, and then lead to new perceptions that emerge between therapist and patient, to be discovered by the patient. As this new quality of experience emerges into language, the process of formulating—finding and creating the words to say it—is itself constitutive of meaning.

Fonagy and his colleagues offer a developmental perspective that revolves around concepts of affect regulation, mentalization, and the development of the self. Mentalization "is the process by which we realise that having a mind mediates our experience of the world".

> We have used the term "reflective function" to refer to our operationalization of the mental capacities that generate mentalization (Fonagy, Gergely, Jurist, & Target, 2004, p. 3)

Mentalized affectivity is the process by which you discover subjective meanings through feeling your feelings. It produces an experiential understanding—I call this *realisation*—beyond the more left-brain, logical, rational, intellectual understanding. How often do patients say "I know this"—but has it been fully realised affectively? For language to complete its job, feelings must mean something that can be formulated through reflection in order to be "communicated to others and interpreted in others to guide collaboration in work, love and play" (Fonagy, Gergely, Jurist, & Target, 2004, p. 6). This capacity for experiential understanding of and embodying the meaning of your emotions ensures "meaningfulness" (2004, p. 15). For young children, however, their mental world can feel real or unreal: "playing with reality, making the real unreal and vice versa, is the principal avenue for the development of mentalization (2004, p. 18). This is perfectly illustrated by what happens when Lucy makes me "pretend" tea.

Lucy gets the last word

As you age, it gets harder to greet every new experience as fresh, to meet the present moment with a first-time ever quality.

What does that have to do with embodied symbolisation? We are talking about what makes life worth living, how meaning is found or created, and how play underpins the creation of symbolic meaning (developed in Part II).

> "Being initiated into language
> is closely connected with playing."
>
> (John M. Heaton)

As I get older, there is nothing that compares with the joyous feeling of a small child coming home, running through the house to find you, leaping into your arms, shrieking with excitement, and then nuzzling into the nape of your neck as you lift them up.

"Look what I got at the zoo!"
"Wow! What is that?"
"It's a baby elephant!"
"Did you see a baby elephant at the zoo?" [*Nodding—I know she loves animals*]
"What else did you see?"
"A tiger, a giraffe, and some monkeys" [*She knows all these words now*]
"Awesome, and who did you go with?"
"Mummy, and Alex and his mum, we had a picnic …"

We can have a proper conversation now. This feels truly miraculous to me. As a parent, I marvelled at my own children's grasping for language, the ability to name things, colours, cars, busses, trains and planes, birds, animals, wind, rain, and thunder. Look! A helicopter! Developing a command of language involves understanding the difference between a picture in a book, a line of text describing it, and the thing itself. Also, it involves understanding the difference between pronouns and nouns, verbs, adverbs, adjectives, and gerunds, similes, metaphors, analogies, the tenses signifying time, and understanding the difference between images, symbols, descriptions, depictions, and allegories. Then, words connect into phrases, sentences, and more complex ideas. Considering the processing involved before a meaningful word can be uttered, it's not surprising some children have difficulties with speech.

"Lucy, do you need to go to the toilet?" She answers "Not yet." She tells me she wants to go back to the beach. I ask: "When did you go there?" And she answers: "Yesterday." I say: "I cannot take you today, but I can take you tomorrow" and she responds: "I want to go now. You take me."

The grasp of time is complex. To speak of "yesterday", "now", and "not yet" with perfect clarity is a mastering of the symbolisation of something abstract. To use the pronouns "I" and "you", and "me" in their right order is impressive. As she goes, she is "getting it" more and more.

Lucy: You didn't take me to the beach but if you come upstairs with me, I will make you tea.
  Me: Okay [*heading to the stairs*], I would love tea, thank you.
       Upstairs, Lucy goes to her doll's house, pulls out the tea set, prepares the tea very carefully and pours me a cup [*the size of my thumb*].
  Me: [*Looking dissatisfied*] But there's no milk in it …
Lucy: [*With astonishment*] USE YOUR IMAGINATION!!

A two-year-old uttering the word "imagination" in context blew me away. Here Lucy was able to move in and out of the play of pretending to make tea seamlessly. It was me that moved out of it, and she brought me back.

> There is evidence that children in their third year who engage more readily in cooperative interaction (Dunn et al. 1991), and specifically in joint pretend play (Astington and Jenkins 1995; Taylor, Gerow, and Carlson 1993; Youngblade and Dunn 1995) show superior mind-reading and emotion understanding performance. (Fonagy, Gergely, Jurist, & Target, 2004, p. 47)

This is a reference to the development of the mentalizing quality of self-organisation (thought to be enhanced by early experience of secure attachment).

To marvel at the achievements of children, to participate, to share the sheer joy, pleasure, and excitement with someone for whom so many of these experiences are *actually* first-time-ever ones, helps to overcome the typical effects of ageing.

If you are sitting around wondering: What is the meaning of life? What is it all for? See the world through the eyes of a two-year-old, see if you can get in touch with your own early experiences of discovery, of both creativity and destructiveness, and of the amazing achievements of development. If you cannot, then share in it with a child. Children are generous, they love to share with you.

If you are not "into" children, or pets, or anything like that—it's okay, of course. You will probably need something or someone "to play with" though if you are to create meaning and grow. And have fun and feel well in the process.

I see all of life as a developmental pathway. There is no expiration date on personal development while you still have a body and language through which to make your life meaning-full.

In Part II we further consider Winnicott's view of early childhood development. The implications for adult development are profound, especially with respect to the importance of play and creativity in meaning-fullness, how meaning is made or found, for both children and adults.

Part II

Play and creativity in child and adult development

CHAPTER 6

The value of illusion

We live in a fantasy world, a world of illusion.
The great task in life is to find reality.
Iris Murdoch

Introduction

The word "illusion" derives from the Latin *illusio* and *illudere*. "Ludere" means "play" and the prefix "il" means "not" or "against". The original meaning of illusion is "not play". This seems counter-intuitive as illusion is a kind of playing in fantasy, but perhaps not playing in reality, as Iris Murdoch indicates.

An example illustrates how the following discussion of illusion in early childhood development applies to adult development and therapy.

During an online session, a bright thirty-five-year-old in another country said that she was happy not to be feeling anxious about the pandemic because "there is so much hysteria when after all it is only really just a cold". It was during the early days, when we were all just learning about coronavirus and its consequences. Feeling I couldn't let that comment pass, I reacted and launched into a rather detailed explanation about pneumonia, lung damage, the ease of transmission, and risks to the already immune-compromised and other aspects of how this virus differed from "just a cold".

My patient texted me later that day, blasting me for making her anxious when she hadn't been, stating it was her prerogative to view the situation as she pleased—without my disillusioning her. A few days later, she texted again saying she was having daily panic attacks.

I emailed and apologised for making her anxious but also said I felt it would have been irresponsible to leave her comment unchallenged.

On reflection, I acted too much like a Covid-19 expert. I said too much—her illusions were smashed—with little preparation. It might have been better to have said "I think it's more than just a cold" or something along the lines of "Seems like you feel safer when you minimise its potential destructiveness" and left it at that, then taking it up further in the next session. The online medium for sessions is difficult and the best approach to discussing the pandemic is debatable. If I had been less challenging, this patient may have left herself unprotected and thereby more susceptible. What if she had then caught Covid-19? And then had infected others? How does illusion have a value and how much disillusionment is the right amount? What kind of play has a value and how is harbouring illusions against play?

Let's look at early childhood development to gain a better understanding of these issues for adults as it is early development that sets the stage for so much of what happens later.

* * *

For early emotional development to go well, there needs to be a comprehensive adaptation by the primary caregiver to the needs of the infant (see Stern, 1998, for more on this). When this is the case, the carer is not perfect but "good-enough". So, if infant is hungry, infant gets fed without undue delay.[36] If baby is cold, baby gets covered up and perhaps held. If baby is anxious or irritable, then baby gets comforted and soothed. Baby's nappy (diaper) is changed as needed and so on. Baby's needs are met in both a practical way and with devotion, care, and love—this is paramount.

While mothering[37] can be efficient in practical ways, some carers are emotionally absent, at least some of the time. Conversely, there are mums who mother with rapport, emotional connectedness, attunement, empathic identification (almost like knowing how it feels to be the baby, this baby), and love, but forget a meal, or leave a dirty nappy too long, and some practicalities are missed. Which would you rather have as a mother? These are not the only possibilities.

---

[36] By "fed" Winnicott means breastfed or bottle-fed but there is also more to it. Good-enough mothering is the total manner or style of mothering on offer. So, popping a breast in the mouth of a hungry baby at the right time is a start but not *enough*. If mum is smoking a cigarette, drinking a beer, and chatting to her friend, or playing games on her phone or watching television, then baby gets fed—but will baby really get nourished in a more complete emotional sense? Good-enough mothering (which is not limited by gender and includes men or anyone offering primary care) involves a high degree of whole-being engagement. This is self-evident to some and escapes others completely.
[37] I am using the term "mother" (and "mothering") in a descriptive sense and as a verb that refers to the actions of mothering in a stereotypical sense (this is socially constructed). This does not exclude men, other women, fathers, grandparents, siblings, friends, or other carers, regardless of gender, age, or relationship, from offering good-enough mothering. Mothering is a role that involves *mothering* actions, not just a position in a kinship relationship.

These days those doing the mothering are busy if not overloaded. Their mothering style will be a mixture of the practical and the emotionally present and connected and will vary both between different carers and for each, depending on how they feel at the time. In other words, some mothers or carers are better than others and some are better some days than other days. Everyone knows this. It is okay to be human, if you can let yourself; along a range of variation, that is *good enough*.

Infants expect mothers to be there, to be responsive and adaptive, to an almost magical degree as if mother was an extension of the baby's own self. This calls to mind our earlier discussion on fusion and merging in adult relationships. Early experiences of merging lead to later feelings of power. Called "early childhood omnipotence", this experience is as if the earth revolves around the child, as if the child is so powerful as to command an all-pervasive influence. It looks very much as if the baby or small child is saying—even prior to the acquisition of language and a more developed sense of self: "If I feel hungry, I expect you to know and feed me—I don't even have to say it in words." Some adults have not grown out of this. Some expect their partners to know how they feel and what they need; they shouldn't have to say. The downside of omnipotence is when everything that goes wrong is felt by children to be their fault because they are so powerful. If a parent is sad and crying (because the stock market went down), children need to be reassured they haven't caused this, neither the event nor mum's reaction to it.

Supporting a sense of omnipotence has value in early care, as the ground of emotional development. But being a good-enough mother does not mean that this level of care must go on indefinitely. As infants grow, and in the normal course of living, there are limits to what can be given. Winnicott calls them "failures" but diminishing adaptation is not a failure. Absolute adaptation to children's desires must wane as they grow older, or they remain children and *fail* to grow up. It can facilitate development for children when parents have a life of their own, independent of their role as parents.

Babies and small children (and big children and adults) need to develop a capacity for frustration, for waiting, for going without, and for not getting exactly what they need or want—right now. If you think about it, probably all of us have failed to get what we needed or thought we needed at some point and survived, maybe even survived perfectly well without it. Often, the frustration of not getting feels worse than the lack of what was needed! Babies and small children need to develop a capacity to cope with a lesser adaptation to their needs gradually and increasingly over time.

Mental activity begins through adaptation to going without, as does a growing sense of process. This means that, in their own way, babies need to develop a capacity to think and understand that when mum leaves the room, she has not disappeared off the face of the earth. She still exists, elsewhere. She will return. And that is okay (for a time)—if baby can cope without excessive anxiety. *If I want to get from A to B, if I want that toy off the shelf, or that book or object, then I will have to get it myself. If I feel anxious and there is no one there to comfort me, then I can grab my teddy and snuggle up and soothe myself.* This is a simple example of what is meant by "the beginnings of mental activity and a sense of process" though no one can say exactly how babies think. Mental activity involves thought, working things out, and process involves a sense of sequence with the passage of time. So, if mum has left the room to speak to someone at the front door, *I can hear they are still talking, they say goodbye, the door closes, footsteps, and she arrives back here*: this is a sequence of events in time.

Thinking and processing involve the development of a sense of space and time. Other examples of process and mental activity are:

1) when dad is preparing food, this involves a sequence of events that occur in time and space, with a beginning, middle, and an end, and results in a meal being served (even if that is warm baby food), and

2) if mum is playing on the floor with baby and rolling a ball back and forth, this occurs in time and space and will ultimately end, perhaps when mum has had enough. The ball has a size and a movement that is affected by the force and direction with which it is rolled. It takes time to reach baby from the moment it leaves mum's hand.

We cannot say *how* babies think or how they understand but we can say that they do think and understand in their own way. When babies and their carers are sufficiently connected, they can often be separated from each other for a time in a non-traumatic way. This is what is meant by the term "secure attachment". It allows those in the parenting role to get on with their work and babies to get on with theirs.

> A secure attachment enables babies to be separated
> and get on with their work as we, the carers and parents,
> get on with ours.

It might seem a strange idea to think of babies working, but babies' learning and development involves a sense of hard work that is ongoing. They are students of everything—of life and of everyone in their field of experience. Work and play are interchangeable in this respect.

The value of illusion

One of the strange contradictions of early childhood development is that infants can gain something essential from parental failures of adaptation to their needs while parents often tend to chastise themselves for these so-called failures. Frustration can make the objects of experience feel real which means objects can be hated as well as loved. The term "objects" here refers to objects of mind which can include things or people, or more accurately the idea of a person. The use of the term "object" in psychoanalytic theory creates confusion because it is often unclear as to whether it refers to a mental object, an object of mind, or a physical object that exists in the world. Object can refer to a person or part of a person, as in part-object. A mental object is better understood as a concept or image.

In adult life, if you ignore me or keep me waiting for a long time (two things I hate) or if you promise to phone me back in ten minutes and then forget, I will start to hate you (even if I love you). It might be for a moment, or longer, but the intense feelings make my idea of you, the mental object or concept, very real to me. Here "real" means there is a power and intensity to my focus upon "you". And, *in reality*, you are not even there.

Comprehensive adaptation[38] to your needs as a small child is rather like magic; the world behaves as you would like, and functions much like a hallucinated wish. To be clear, at the very start, maternal adaptation to need must be comprehensive, or close to it, to form a basis, a foundation, for the experience of reality—as something beyond oneself—and a capacity to form a conception of it and to recognise your conception as such. There is a curious paradox at play. A baby while completely helpless and dependent grows to feel omnipotent[39]—all powerful—for the beginnings of a sense of self to be possible. Without self, there can be no sense of difference— different to what? This is often referred to as "external reality" but it is not a matter of external-ity, it is a matter of difference or otherness, and the development of an identity depends on an experience and an emerging concept of difference. *And this is where illusion comes in.*

In the beginning, world and self are *as if* one, theoretically. By virtue of adaptation to need, good-enough mothering allows the infant the illusion that the world is controlled by the infant (as if magic). From the baby's point of view (though not articulated as such), I think it, or I want it, or I need it, and so it is there, presented to me, as if wanting creates having, hav-ing follows wanting. Development involves a movement through omnipotence in which desire and having are merged, to disillusionment in which the dialectic of desire emerges. When hav-ing and wanting are dialectically related, they are first disentangled as two separate "things" in opposition such that you cannot have what you want because once you have it, desire is sated. The synthesis of the two allows for a sense of satisfaction in having what you want, important in the capacity to sustain relationships and personal connections over time.

Omnipotence characterises early experience, especially of desire. The task of good-enough parenting, of helping children to grow up emotionally, is one of gradual and gentle, disil-lusionment involving the recognition of otherness as distinct from self. In the process, a

---

[38] Many mothers who suffer post-natal depression (PND) feel a profound sense of shame (to a paralysing degree) because of their perceived *inability* to respond to their new baby with a nearly total adaptation to their baby's needs and yet they know this is what is required of them, and they expect it of themselves. At its worst, PND pre-vents mothers from responding or functioning which makes it worse, self-determining, and self-perpetuating—a proverbial vicious cycle.

[39] Omnipotence tends to develop around two years old, though it varies.

growing recognition of self emerges, again essential for relationships that work. *First, illusion, then disillusionment.*

In adult psychotherapy, the task of disillusionment is often still unfinished.[40] Winnicott's ideas relate to adults in much the same way as to young children. For my patient in the example at the beginning of this chapter, ideally there would be more time for gradual disillusionment, much as small children need to give up illusions. For psychotherapy to be developmental, we need to understand the role of disillusionment.

> Calvin was a stay-at-home Dad who looked after his three-year-old while his wife, Maddie, worked as a barrister. In couples therapy, Maddie complained that Calvin was often spaced-out, forgot to do tasks; he even forgot to collect their son from day care.
>
> Even when Maddie was home, he seemed preoccupied with something or other, he had his face in the computer. He was working on something though it was never clear what or how it would be of value. She felt unsupported.
>
> Having explored this over some time, I proposed to Calvin that he was a rock star waiting to be discovered. He didn't play a musical instrument, but what I meant by this comment was that he was operating under a fantasy—an illusion—of fame, or of being someone who would accomplish great things. He was wondering when the world would notice and celebrate him. All this was going on in his mind, in a private place in himself. Calvin knew exactly what I meant though Maddie was shocked. She had no idea.

Illusion has a value for child development but becomes an obstacle to development, and to living, if not overcome in adulthood.

Many adults are still holding out for life to give them what they want because they want it (and now, please). With that said, I think that a certain measure of illusion, of hope, of faith, that the future will be better, and you will get something of what you want before too long, is desirable. It can prevent depression, or act as an antidote to an existing depression. Depression is many things but usually there is a sense of loss and a bleak outlook towards the future. Disillusionment can go too far or perhaps too fast, as it did for my patient who thought the coronavirus was *just* a cold, another example of how being right is not always helpful.

> ## Being right in principle can mean being wrong in therapy.

* * *

---

[40] A friend told me that he complained to his therapist that he was feeling disillusioned, and his therapist replied: "Why would you want to live in illusion?"

Notice the difference between what is there to be perceived (that is, how things appear in themselves) and your own subjective conception of these very things, what you make of them, in your way of apprehending them, from your point of view. This is the difference between perception and conception, perception of the world and conception in your way of thinking about it. Of course, your perceptions are subjective and informed by your conceptions, but this is what I want to sort out. Try to see things as they are, and notice how your conception, your agenda, your desire affects your perceptions. There is a transition from omnipotence, by which you see things mainly in terms of how you want them to be (narcissism) to a phenomenological[41] attitude, by which you see things as they are or as close to "reality" as possible, even if objectivity is never fully achievable. This can involve a clarity of vision that takes account of your own personal filters, your subjective lens, your point of view, and your personal way of looking at things, your perspective, and biases. You cannot be fully objective, but objectivity is your objective, the direction to be moving towards. The closer you get to objectivity, the more you have succeeded in overcoming omnipotence, repudiating the vestiges of childhood, and transcending your individual, subjective position. This is what Frankl called "self-transcendence". The idea of transitional experience in the development of self-transcendence is explored in detail as we go and especially through the long psychotherapy case of Luke in Part IV.

Adult development involves growing from a schizoid quality of experience which is largely informed by fantasy to something like the Heideggerian *being-in-the-world* where there can be no sense of self separate from the world that situates you, and no sense of world without you as a part of it (while alive). Even in the translation of this formulation of being-*in*-the world, the word *in* appears, but the hyphens indicate that what *is* cannot be separated from the world it is *in*. It's not that there is "no separation"—self and world are not the same, it's not a fusion—rather, you cannot have a self without a world, and you cannot have a world without the selves that populate it. *World* is not a container in which we are situated. The term "world" refers more to our total context-in-the-flow-of-time. It is not a static "thing". Ultimately, the duality of what is felt to be inside you and perceived as outside of you, between concept and world, needs to be overcome. Heidegger's great work *Being and Time* (1962) is an ontological analysis of the meaning of being, something he believed had been missed by the Western metaphysical tradition of philosophy.

The point of discussing development as a movement from split-experiencing (living in your head—as Calvin was—or, as some people describe it, living from behind their eyes) to

---

[41] Phenomenology is a philosophical attitude that privileges description of experience over explanation. For me, the best introduction to phenomenology is Maurice Merleau-Ponty's Preface to *The Phenomenology of Perception* (1962, pp. vii–xxi) in which he calls it a descriptive psychology. Phenomenology is the philosophical underpinning of my approach to psychotherapy. I couldn't possibly call my practice psychoanalytic phenomenology or, worse, existential/phenomenological/psychoanalytic/developmental psychotherapy. (A marketing nightmare!)

integrated experiencing (self as part of world, world as part of self) is that this very movement is evident in both child development and the developmental gains of adults in psychotherapy. This is one meaning of the oft-used term "integration". Integration also means being fully involved or absorbed in what you are doing while still retaining a separate sense of self, not-fused; emotionally engaged while retaining your identity. The most common usage of "integration" refers to the disparate parts of a person being connected to one another, and not dis-integrated (or dissociated). But integration should also refer to significant others, as no person is an island, no matter how isolated or split-off.

Winnicott is advocating a clear space, a neutral zone of experience, a transitional space, and what he also calls an intermediate area of experience, for this developmental movement to be facilitated. This is vital for early childhood development just as it is for adult development in psychotherapy. The problem with calling it an intermediate area is that we revert to the use of a spatial metaphor that involves an inside and an outside. And it is that very split that needs to be overcome.

Notice the use of spatial metaphors above: space, zone, area—it is difficult to speak of what is meant without using them (even for Heidegger!). Calvin, for example, is stuck in an interior mental space in himself and needs to get out of his head and into the world. There is no literal space inside him that he is *in*. Equally, saying "into the world" does not mean into something spatial, it means "involved". He needs to engage directly in his life, his responsibilities, his tasks, with his son and partner. The transition is from withdrawn and mentally and emotionally absent (or, at least partially) to connected, attuned, with-it, on-the-ball, attentive—in a word, engaged. If he can do that, he will promote his son's early development better and his wife will be happier with him. Couples therapy can be developmental.

In an everyday sense, we come upon people to whom something greatly matters. They may be fixed on a particular issue or cause or pursuit. It forms the core of their discourse, what they most want to talk about, think about, and maybe even (try to) convince you to enlist. In understanding the value of transitional experience, this *mattering* is not challenged. As a therapist or friend or lover or stranger, whatever you think of it, however much you doubt its value, even if you think it is completely mistaken, it is left to the person to hold in their own way. This is what "non-judgemental" refers to in therapy. One day they may grow towards disillusionment and thereby lose interest (to your relief) but this happens in their own way, in their own time, if left unchallenged. Some causes are worth dying for. That said, a virus isn't one of them, and there are other exceptions such as the sorts of illusions that leave patients (and others) in the path of harm. An example would be the person who thinks that protection is unnecessary in sex because they will never catch a sexually transmitted infection. There are many examples of bizarre beliefs.

Calvin did hold a passionate conviction about a political cause—that was not challenged. He struggled to do anything about it, to serve the cause in meaningful ways. I did gently challenge his struggle by saying he would probably feel better, more fulfilled, if he could embark on small contributions instead of waiting to be elected Prime Minister.

My patient from Chapter 5 needed one session. I never said anything about, nor had to confirm or disconfirm, her strong conviction of a literal frog *in* her physical throat. Rather, we attended to what that meant to her, the intentional meaning as opposed to the referential meaning. She had made another appointment but then cancelled it. When she phoned me, she said her voice was fine now and I could hear that it was. She realised that not telling her husband her feelings was making her ill, and she told him that. She realised she needed to tell him how she felt in a non-confrontational and unprovocative way. Then, he could hear it and, she told me, he was more receptive. She didn't want or need long-term therapy, but I would still like to call her one session *developmental*, at least potentially.

A confrontation instigates opposition in the form of a fight, an argument, resistance, and protest and rarely, if ever, succeeds in prompting disillusionment. This applies to mental health practices, too. Some practitioners confront what they consider errors in your thinking. You are depressed because you think you are worthless. They will show you how many ways you are *really* worthy, so you can think of yourself differently and so no longer feel depressed. I've been told many times that patients became convinced the psychologist didn't *really* recognise them. They already knew what they had going for them but still felt worthless. Alternatively, it is easy to become dependent on a professional authority convinced of your worth and attempting to bolster your sense of self-esteem.

The idea of low self-esteem is a relatively recent invention with many consequences.

> In the last 20 years of so there has been an enormous increase in the number of experts in the management of individual psychology especially emotion (Ferudi, 2004). To give one statistic, in 1980 there was no reference to "self-esteem" in 300 UK newspapers. By 1990 the figure was 103. And by 2000 there was a staggering 3,328 references to it (Ferudi, 2004: 2–4). A low level of self-esteem is associated with a huge range of problems from crime to teenage pregnancy. As self-esteem is such a vague concept pretty well anyone can be made to feel they have this diagnosis. This opens the way to seeking professional help who then exercise control by normalising the sick role, encouraging us to seek identity through a diagnosis, so promoting the virtue of dependence on professional authority. (Heaton, 2006, p. 57)

Thinking you are worthless or "have" low self-esteem, a common belief, is complicated. The illusion here is created out of an abstraction of "self"—the idea or concept of self as worthless, or even simply "lesser". It is a global generalisation (what Levinas (1969) called "totalizing") founded upon nothing of substance—there is no criterion to assess worth—and hence the notion is "abstracted", removed from the world. It is a purely mental construct. It raises questions about how a self is valued and how a person's worth can be measured or determined. How does a person come to feel better about their sense of self-worth? Such pathogenic beliefs need to be dismantled to free up energy to work towards self-improvement if self-improvement is even what is needed. Isn't it an illusion to think that a "self" even has a "worth" other than what you mean *to someone* at a particular point in time? The preoccupation with self-worth in the abstract is a formula to get you down because there is no register to determine it.

If the illusion of worthlessness has any value at all, it resides in the way it provides a rationalisation for not trying or achieving (or "good-enough achieving" because, ironically, many *worthless* people are high achievers). It also provides a developmental opportunity to grow out of this negative preoccupation with self and get into the world and do something of value, even if only in a small way. While doing something of value is a great antidote for worthlessness, there is also a value in getting on with your life and living it—if you can—as you are. This is part of mental health, as I see it: realising no one is worthless and no one is worth everything. Comparing and contrasting oneself negatively to others doesn't work. It is an imaginary exercise that results in self defeat. You can always find someone better, smarter, richer, more beautiful, more accomplished, or superior in whatever register, if you look—or the opposite—if you look in the other direction. It turns being a person into a competition with others.

One of the great benefits of working as a psychotherapist is that in listening to someone else, you forget your self-preoccupation, replace it with other-occupation, and invariably feel better.

Challenging, disproving, or disputing the illusion—whatever form it takes—does not facilitate development. That requires a therapeutic process. When I said to Calvin "You are a rock star", I didn't say "You have the illusion of being a rock star", or "You shouldn't see yourself that way". Believing you are a rock star when not a rock star, like a short circuit, describes a state of waiting, a latency, hence Calvin's passivity and mental/emotional absence. He is absent because he is present to his own mental preoccupations with his value, his potential achievements, his imagined recognition for that, and his pride at being a beacon of light, a hero, a star (in fantasy). I invited him to challenge himself about this, and thereby disillusion himself.

A therapeutic process that promotes disillusionment is like the graduated weaning of a small child from breastfeeding. We are not just talking about a measured decrease of a purely practical nature, like turning down the volume control. The experience of weaning for the young child and how this is felt, as it unfolds, needs to be considered.

- How does the child handle the change in attitude from the mother?
- How is frustration managed?
- How does the child cope with *no*, with mum reclaiming her body as her own?
- How does the child react to mum's refusal?
- Is there room for negotiation between them?

Weaning needs to be negotiated. There is give and take on both sides.[42] There is no need to make an issue of it when it goes well enough. It is a process of illusion/disillusionment, of omnipotence reduction, of mediated narcissism reduction, and of the development of a capacity to go without. Just stopping is not a weaning; it is cold turkey. (Note: the relevance to adult addictions.)

With the completion of weaning there is a more complete sense of separation between the body of the mother and the body of the child. This is a continuous process from conception, through gestation, birth, and the earliest parent–infant bond expressed in holding, warming, feeding, and soothing to being a separate person. Baby is becoming physically separate and psychologically separate in parallel processes. And this usually continues as baby grows older and grows up. Held less, with fewer hugs, kisses, and caresses, most of us move towards the more formal physical contact of two adults who are not lovers. A relationship forms between two *separate* individuals. You can still hug.

If you recall Steph from Chapter 4, Jake withdrew abruptly from the relationship with her. There was no weaning. She couldn't cope with that and wanted to kill herself. It was not only like a death *to* her but the death *of* her. She needed time and a process of coming to terms with it—a form of adult weaning—but he didn't give her that. The two weeks in hospital was just enough. Many couples have a kind of to-and-fro movement of separating, coming back together and moving apart on the way to a more final separation. This is a kind of weaning.

There are other examples. We can become attached, if not addicted, to all kinds of things, ideas, and goals. The hardest thing is to let go all at once. The letting go of something you want so badly—my football team's winning the Grand Final—is also a process of illusion giving way to disillusionment (especially in the case of my football team!). How this is negotiated makes all the difference to how painful the process is. It helps if other people understand and support the process.

Part of growing up and, if you're lucky, growing old, involves a giving up of the illusions around a glorious future, an idea you may have held with great hope and conviction. Another part is weaning yourself from your dependence upon your parents. That means emotionally and financially. It doesn't mean you can't be close. Often, when children grow up and have their own children, their parents become more involved again—but in a different way. When parents want to be the boss of the grandchildren and the experts on how they are raised, conflict tends to ensue. In such cases, the grandparents haven't sufficiently weaned from their role as parents. Grandparenting works better if the children, now the parents of the grandchildren, determine

---

[42] In unhurried weaning, often a child will slowly initiate self-weaning, as they feel ready to go without the former frequency and regularity of breastfeeding. Mother may well feel a greater sense of loss than the child. In her classic article, Erna Furman (1982) challenged Kleinian assumptions that weaning is always a loss for the child.

how they are raised—which will be different. (I've learned a lot from watching my children become parents.)

In one example from my practice, a patient told me his parents referred to his daughters in different ways that indicated the children *belonged* to his parents, the *grandparents*. "How are my girls today? It's lovely to have daughters now. I'm so looking forward to seeing my kids." And so on. My patient felt increasingly uncomfortable at a competitiveness creeping in from his parents. He also appreciated their involvement and support, as he was on his own, had the girls full time and worked full time.

Getting the balance right between separateness and connectedness can be a challenge. For example, do you feel completely separate from your parents? If you complete the journey of growing up and developing into an adult, does that mean that you are one hundred per cent separate from your parents? Or if/when your children grow up, are they totally separate from you? How separate should they be from you? Or you from them? How separate do you want them to be? How separate do you want your parents to be? You can have no contact with your parents and still not be separate from them. Your "parents" dwell in your psyche through your concept of them, "your internal objects".

It is very hard to answer these questions with precision, and the answers won't be the same for everyone. Some people can't get far enough away from their parents! And based on what I've heard of parental mistreatment and worse, abuse—fair enough, too—and vice versa. Even in these circumstances, can you be completely separate? How many times have I heard: "Though they abused me, I still love them?" Okay, but are you separate enough?

In a different sort of example, imagine that you sit next to someone on a New York subway train, and then at the next stop everyone gets off except the person sitting next to you. When the train departs, they get up and move diagonally to the far end of the carriage. Would you wonder why? I would. Why did they get as far away from me as possible? Do I have body odour? *Don't they like me?* This action must have something to do with me. Wouldn't you wonder? Or would you just drop it? There's nothing in it. Just a stranger—who cares? How long would you dwell on it? Minutes, hours, days, months? (This happened to me over fifty years ago and I'm still wondering). How separate are we?

> Even total strangers are connected in a way that can easily feel too much or too little.

From conception to death, living is a developmental journey through transitional experiencing. This process involves the perpetual movement from illusion to disillusion and separating-out of self from other. It is essential to the capacity to connect and have a meaningful relationship and to gaining an understanding of who you are to someone and who they are to you.

A: You love me?

B: Yes.

A: Why do you love me?

B: I don't know, I just do.

A: Yeah, but there must be a reason.

B: I suppose.

A: So, what do you love about me?

B: I love the way you wrinkle up your nose when you smile.

A: [*Dissatisfied*] So, you love me because of how I look?

B: No, there are lots of things I love about you but what do you want, do you want me to list them?

A: Sure, go on then, I want to know. I want to understand it.

B: [*Getting annoyed*] I don't have a list; I love the way you make me feel.

A: So, I stroke your ego and you love that.

B: [*More annoyed*] Look, I don't think there is anything I can say that will satisfy you so why don't you just drop it.

A: I'm starting to doubt that you really do love me.

B: Okay, I don't love you, besides I'm sick of this.

A: [*Crying*] I knew it, that's why I was asking, I knew it.

B: Oh my God … I didn't mean it.

Here, A is putting pressure on B, A's partner, attempting an intellectual analysis of B's love, much to B's annoyance. It only takes a moment to destroy it. Love has a quality of illusion in the sense discussed here. I'm not saying that love isn't real. It hangs on a belief, a feeling, a cultural construction, all of which is subject to being destroyed under enough pressure. If I value something and I call it *love*—I love my wife, I love my children, I love my work, I love my home—I don't want anyone calling any of this into question. Who are you to analyse my love?

- Can I prove my love?
- Will it stand up to scientific scrutiny?
- Research studies?
- Will it survive psychoanalytic analysis?
- Or could it be damaged by the disapproval of those in authority, or my family or friends?
- Should I change my thinking because a professional person says so?

Destruction happens all too easily. This is also why disillusion also needs to be left to the timing of each person's own developmental process. Then, if there is loss, it belongs to you and is not caused by someone else. The disillusionment is your own and the corresponding disorientation and adjustment needed are free to happen without resentful feelings of having been pushed, directed, or manipulated. You are free to grieve and move on. Therapy needs to cast sunlight into the darkness, without gaslight[43] along the way.

The intermediate or neutral zone of experience needs to be a protected space, safe, private, and unassailable. It is the "place" where a transitional object can appear, where transitional experiencing can allow the gradual movement towards disillusionment. This occurs early on for children (when does a teddy become *just* a teddy?) and as a parallel process later on for adults. Protecting this "space" or process is a task for anyone involved who understands it. Many people have their childhood teddies on their adult pillows.

Transitional experiencing is the stage on which the play of development unfolds. It is the condition of the possibility, the breeding ground for meaning and purpose to emerge, through attention and care, and affording the opportunity of illusion that is available throughout life and belongs to intense, affective living. This underscores the possibility of meaningful living and is its source. Disillusionment does not have to be total or absolute. There is a value in illusion, to a degree and for a time. It serves a developmental function that is furthered by disillusionment.

I have a little pond with fish outside. I talk to them. I pretend they talk back to me. It's a little eccentric, I know. It's play. I like them. They come to greet me when I appear (okay, they know I am feeding them). We have a mutually rewarding relationship. We enjoy each other's company. Is this an illusion? A real relationship? Or a symptom of a mental disorder?

* * *

Coming to terms[44] with "reality", overcoming omnipotence, weaning off your illusions as you grow up, becoming more separate as a person, and forming an authentic identity, are all elements of a developmental process that goes on throughout your adult life, and is a movement towards mental health. This process is more burdensome for some who, through no fault of their own, have not achieved the proper foundations in their early development. Quite possibly, no one is to blame. Life does not provide ideal conditions for growing up. The strain of this burden can be mitigated by people who are sympathetic, understanding, and supportive. Psychotherapy may be needed. Meditation helps. Yoga is beneficial. And my personal favourite: I place a high therapeutic value on the power of music and dance. Opportunities for the creative potential of play should be maximised in this context.

---

[43] The contemporary term "gaslighting" comes from the play *Gaslight* which was made into a film in the 1940s. The character played by Charles Boyer manipulated the character played by Ingrid Bergman by changing the lighting in her living space, while claiming with faux innocence that nothing had changed. Gaslighting occurs when a version of reality is constructed, often with deliberate distortion, and then is imposed, as the gaslighter sets out to convince you that your version of reality is wrong. You could be made to feel crazy in the process. This can apply to children or adults equally.

[44] In the double-sense I indicated before in relation to symbolisation—acceptance and coming to language.

Some people find that they cannot come to terms with "reality" because of the lack of essential capacities. Relief may be found, however, by the cultivation of transitional experience that is in direct continuity with the play space of the small child. Play, getting lost in play, the intense experiencing of play, play that can feel like a matter of life and death, provides opportunities for reconciling your experiences of self and world, and overcoming the dualities of inner and outer, real and unreal, and self and others.

In a sense, play affords opportunities to move from illusion to disillusion. Play also informs attitudes in your relation to work, love, sex, God/spirit, money, relationships, and even living itself. The value of illusion finds its greatest fulfilment in the way play leads to the realisation of your creative potential to make meaning and to create something of value.

> Living tilts from struggle to an art form
> on the fulcrum of play.

CHAPTER 7

Work and play

Children learn as they play.
Most importantly, in play
children learn how to learn.
O. Fred Donaldson

A patient in psychotherapy had a lightbulb moment. He realised he had always made work and career his primary reference and priority. How should he spend his time? What should he do next? Would whatever he did further the development of his work and career? Of course, his partner and children mattered too—but he rationalised that the more his ambitions were fulfilled, the better he could support his family. Everything was filtered through this lens. What he realised was that there was no place for how he felt at any given moment to have a part in this process. Feelings didn't come into it. When he finally managed to combine work with his emotional life, he became more centred in himself, his values, and what mattered most in the moment. He was happier, more relaxed, balanced, and the quality of his relationships was enhanced. While work and career remained important, he had no sense that he was any less productive or successful. Work informed by feelings created a shift to a lighter and more playful approach to life; he felt more emotionally available, too, and less worn-out.

This striking transformation helps further the consideration of play raised in the previous chapter. At a glance, the difference between work and play may seem obvious. Play is fun, brings pleasure, excitement, and enjoyment. You feel alive and engaged. Work, by contrast, is what *has to* be done. It has its rewards but at its worst, it can feel deadly, dull, routine, and utterly boring—a grind, serving time as a survival strategy. For many, living is skewed towards what *has to* be done rather than what *wants to* be done. Accordingly, play becomes an "antidote" to the struggle of living.

The following discussion takes a different approach. When considered more fully, the opposition between work and play is less obvious and less reducible to contrasting activities. There is overlap and interplay, and the line of demarcation blurs. In this context, the role of play is significant. The film *Life is Beautiful* (1997) comes to mind. The main character turns war into play to protect his young son from its horrors. This works as distraction for a child. For adults, such as the patient with the lightbulb moment, play in the broadest sense *integrates* what *has* to be done with what *wants* to be done. This chapter suggests that play is valuable for therapy and explores its implications for meaning, creativity, and a life worth living.

Work

I want to focus on a particular idea of work which has emerged as a cultural dominant in recent times under the pervasive forces of late capitalism: the obsessive concern with productivity. Let me set the scene.

When I went to university and did my undergraduate degree in the early 1970s, there was an emphasis on learning for its own sake. We were encouraged to study subjects of interest, those that would make us informed but, more so, thoughtful, and would help us gain understanding and intellectual experience. We were encouraged to think critically but not taught what to think. One highlight was studying philosophy of education taught by the university president in his lounge room, in the evening in front of an open fire, while sipping Irish coffees. It made learning such a pleasure. In the liberal arts, learning was developmental, there was no set goal to be reached or outcome to be achieved. There were no competencies to be assessed. We were not being groomed for a particular job or career, industry, or profession. We were being educated in learning how to learn through the development of personal resources for living which includes working. Some of the values espoused throughout this book arise from that early influence.

By contrast, universities today seem akin to degree factories. Education, so-called, has become the mass production of a skilled workforce (though some come through more skilled than others), overly focused on productive outcomes at the expense of personal development. You are lucky if your occasional tutor turns up. Care for students' emotional needs is almost non-existent. Education appears to be about getting a job, training for a career, and being able to apply what you've learned when you enter the workforce, such as to produce something, and fast (as measured by Key Performance Indicators). It also resembles a profit-driven business, like most big corporations. Leverage everything, cram as many students as possible into a lecture theatre and put all study material online. It is the students' responsibility to educate themselves, and personal contact, mentoring, and attention to the detail of students' work is compromised, sometimes out of existence. There are no Irish coffees now.

This shift is pervasive in contemporary culture, which has moved towards an emphasis—indeed, an obsession—with work as sheer productivity. I see a general trend of people working harder, for longer, and for less than ever before. I am all for work and have been fortunate to have had a solid career of it. I also see consequences in people getting more and more tired, run down, disheartened, and demoralised, or worse still: burnt out.[45] This seems to be the new normal and I hear it in my consulting room more often. The intensification of pressure to be productive comes at the expense of being, at the expense of physical and emotional health, and consequently at the expense of some of the most fundamental questions of what it means to be a person:

1. Who am I?
2. What do I want?
3. Where am I going?
4. What really matters?
5. What is my life for?

Difficulty answering is common in psychotherapy practice though sessions are a good opportunity to consider such questions. Becoming busier and busier, sometimes frantic with busyness, overloaded with demands, commitments, obligations, and deadlines, leads to an increase in worry, stress, fear, and panic—often building up to anxiety, depression, burn-out, and worse, the risk of breakdown. Referring to work or even their way of living in general, people often say "I don't know why I'm doing this, all I know is living is hectic". There is a feeling of running a race but not knowing why or where the finish line is. Even if you are getting somewhere desirable such as increasing your overall net worth in financial terms, there is often a feeling that the cost outweighs the benefit—no matter how desirable the benefit—and the cost is felt in its compromise of both mental and physical health, not to mention relationships. Throughout his life, one man said "It will all be worth it when we retire". Then, his wife died at forty-eight years old. His entire paradigm for living broke down and he wound up in mental hospital. He had electro-convulsive shock therapy for a "major depressive episode". When he got out, he went back to work in the same way. After a further twenty years, he retired at sixty-five years old but then had ten years of terrible depression because he didn't know what to live for without his work. Then he died. That was my father and his wife, my mother.

Clinically, I have often heard despair expressed as "I worked my butt off for my family, did the hard yards, built a substantial estate, and we have lived a fabulous lifestyle, but I suppose, in the end, it cost me my marriage and family. I didn't have enough time to give the relationship to make it work and for my partner to feel valued. If anything, my partner pleaded with me to put a brake on it and put some limits and boundaries in place, spend more time together and with the kids, and have more fun. But there was always this pressure to keep pushing-on even though I could see everything being eroded at the same time." This is regrettable.

---

[45] "Burn-out" is now classified as an "occupational phenomenon" in ICD-11 from chronic workplace stress as the World Health Organisation is working on evidence-based guidelines for mental well-being in the workplace.

Transitional experiencing, a sense of exchange between self and world, and play underlying creativity, are all reaching towards a more authentic way of living in balance, optimising possibilities for meaning-fullness. The excessive emphasis on productivity leads towards a more compliant, doing-what-you-have-to-or-are-supposed-to-do way of living. It motivates taking on too much debt and then finding yourself *having to* keep on producing to keep head above water. Now you are on a treadmill that is very hard to get off without sacrifice and a radical reduction in lifestyle. This downward adjustment is one that people typically find painful and humiliating. Excess debt is also toxic. The associated stress and related feelings often lead to compensatory practices like overeating, excessive drinking, drug binges, overspending, chasing sex, gambling, and other sorts of gratifications pursued in a compulsive way. Do you find you need to seek compensation for your efforts?

I've learned, by getting it wrong myself, that it is better to live at a standard below the very top of what you might be able to afford if you were to work all hours and borrowed to the hilt to manage it. It is better to have time for being, for doing things for their own sake, and for the things and people that matter—even though they won't make for a bigger house, a fancier car, or a holiday in Bora Bora. Your relationship in the smaller house will be more loving and satisfying, which will make most people happier than watching your joint estate get divided because of separation and divorce with all the associated costs. Everything you were working for was to prevent that: to live together and perhaps raise kids together, to live well towards an open-ended and harmonious future. Happily ever after. If not forever, at least ongoingly. And what cost is incurred in the quality of parenting and children's overall experience of their childhoods as they get older. The way you live is the model of living you reflect to your kids who are growing up to live as adults. Like you? The way you feel reflects to your kids the effect of your way of living and working. How will they feel when they grow up? Should they follow your modelling or the opposite. What is the emotional cost? What developmental cost? It is unquantifiable. There is no metric. No survey or questionnaire can tell you. Even though it can't be counted, it still counts.

In this context, it is valuable to put pressure on the notion of productivity. Aristotle divided human activity into three basic categories: *theoria* or thinking, *poiesis* or making (not poetry), and *praxis* or doing. He discusses the relation between praxis and theoria— the putting into practice what has been thought. Thus Marx: "Practice without theory is blind. Theory without practice is sterile" (from memory). In this case, however, I am interested in the relation between praxis and productivity. The actual distinction I want to make is technically between autotelic praxis, the purpose or existence of which comes from within itself, and heterotelic praxis ("telic" refers to telos: meaning aim or goal) where the purpose of the action comes from outside itself. Here, I refer to autotelic praxis as praxis-for-its-own-sake and heterotelic praxis as praxis-for-the-sake-of-sheer productivity. It is an imperfect distinction, but I see a value in applying it to contemporary living. It will help to consider examples.

Praxis-for-its-own-sake

Examples are play in general, meditation, making music, sport, yoga, painting, walking, swimming, taking your child to the park or playground, reading a novel, watching TV or a movie, and, let's not forget: loving. You might seek to develop your ability and work towards excellence, or *eupraxis*—but you don't have to. Examples of praxis-for-its-own-sake also exist in excellence of character such as fairness, integrity, courage, in ethical virtues such as honesty, trustworthiness, wisdom, and in well-being such as the ways that friendship, camaraderie, closeness, engagement, involvement, and connectedness with others can make you feel well and happy. What makes you most happy? Is it the sorts of activities above or when you are most productive? It could be both, but there is a different feeling associated with each. When I am productive, I tend to feel relief, sometimes pride, or pleasure, perhaps even fulfilled if it refers to something I really wanted to get done (like this book!) When I am immersed in making music or sport or walking in the forest or loving my loved ones, I feel a different quality of happiness. I feel more fulfilled as a person, a whole person, by virtue of the inherent meaning and value in this sense of praxis.

Praxis-for-the-sake-of-sheer-productivity

Sheer productivity differs in that there is an end goal or purpose in producing something external to the action involved. In productivity, you produce something whereas in praxis-for-its-own-sake, the actions involve internal reasons for doing so. The activity of sheer productivity is directed towards achieving this pre-determined goal; the activity itself is a means to an end. Satisfaction is gained as much from external approval or recognition as your own inner sense of achievement. As I noted earlier, our society is skewed towards sheer productivity, with consequences that are both rife and dire, not least for mental health.

If you want to accomplish anything, then you probably have to work in the productive mode. Work hard if you want to get anywhere in this world, there is no substitute for it. If you want to be successful, specialise. Become better, more knowledgeable, more effective, and become known in a smaller field than if you are "horizontal" and know quite a lot along a wide spectrum. Become the best in a narrowly defined area. Start early and apply yourself. Innovate. Think outside the box (or better, make the box larger). Do it your way instead of being rule-bound and restricted (think: Steve Jobs). There is no shortage of memes full of good advice for being successful.

Let's not forget what you are doing it for. Let's not forget to have a life along the way. Otherwise, your creativity becomes confined to the productive, while the best, most meaningful rewards of your creativity—the intangibles—are lost. Both modes of praxis are important: training for a career and learning and gaining knowledge. However, the contemporary focus on productive outcomes is frequently at the expense of personal development. The psychotherapy clinic sees more people who are good at their jobs, competent, but not happy, not sure if what they're doing is right for them and feeling negative inside (in different ways). Their relation to their work is conflicted, often ambivalent. I hear these sorts of comments regularly:

- "I'm not sure I'm in the right place."
- "I feel a bit of my soul being destroyed each day."
- "My working life is full of cognitive dissonance."
- "I love being good at what I do and commanding a high salary, but I hate that it means nothing to me."
- "I don't care about the company I work for."
- "I've never worked so hard, my days are getting longer."
- "Now I take work home in the evenings and on the weekends."
- "I am going backwards financially even though I have never earned this much money before or worked this hard."

Surely, we need to look at this. Speaking of emotional development, Winnicott wrote: "'I am' must precede 'I do', otherwise 'I do' has no meaning for the individual" (1971, p. 130). Through such comments, ontology meets psychoanalysis. For doing to be meaningful, first there needs to be a "self" and the "self" needs to be grounded in a capacity for "being". The more you develop a sense of self, the more you know why you are doing what you're doing and the more you want to do it for its own sake—or you change it. Also, the more your sense of self grows organically as an authentic expression of your identity rather than a socially constructed "self" that fears slipping out of the mould and hence becomes self-consciously fearful of censure and critical commentary. A greater sense of self arises and grows out of play.

Play

Play facilitates emotional growth and development towards emotional health. I have discussed the importance of play for children. It is equally important for adults and has a vital role in making the psychotherapy of adults into a developmental process. Winnicott's statement on playing and psychotherapy has changed the way many therapists view what they do.

> *Psychotherapy takes place in the overlap of two areas of playing, that of the patient and that of the therapist. Psychotherapy has to do with two people playing together. The corollary of this is that where playing is not possible then the work done by the therapist is directed towards bringing the patient from a state of not being able to play into a state of being able to play.* (1971, p. 38, original emphasis)

Here I have changed Winnicott's construction into something more generalised:

Life takes place in the overlap of two areas of playing, that of the self and that of the world. The corollary of this is that where playing is not possible, then the work needed is directed towards bringing ourselves from a state of not being able to play into a state of being able to play.

Where possible, playing can make even the most unbearable situation bearable (for example, the film *Life is Beautiful* (1997)).

There is nothing frivolous in using play in therapy or, indeed, living. Viewing psychotherapy as play shifts the emphasis from the serious business of treating mental disorders, though that remains, to a greater emphasis on feeling well and happy, enjoyment, and creating greater ease by a change in attitude and orientation to living. It puts the serious work of psychotherapy in a different light, a lighter light, without diminishing the seriousness of the work at once. In some ways, the more serious the condition, the greater the need for a lighter approach—an apparent contradiction, no doubt.

Consider the implications for those suffering from emptiness and meaninglessness. Some of pain's intensity is relieved when looked at differently. Of course, the world doesn't exist to provide you with joy, meaning, and other rewards—you don't get frequent flyer points for each trip around the sun—yet there is *something* there for you, if you can engage in interplay with the world and the possibilities it offers.

This becomes even more important as conditions worsen. Over the course of my lifetime, in many parts of the world, conditions for living have deteriorated. We can expect that trend to continue, unfortunately. This qualification is needed: there is more to mental health than a shift of attitude. The orientation and attitude towards play is only one aspect, albeit an important one.

For children, playing is far more conducive when the environment lends itself to playing and that includes the carers' attitude and participation in the children's playing—*their* playing. Are there things to play with? Are there objects that stimulate the senses? Colourful, noisy, or musical objects, and bright with child-like imagery that tweaks the imagination? Things, activities, experiences give children choices. The same questions can be applied to adults of all ages. Are there adults to play with who are truly playful? Colourful, noisy, bright, stimulating adults with whom to engage in play. Why should we have less fun as we get older?

The process of play in the earliest stages involves an interplay between omnipotence—referring to the baby's (apparent) belief in the ownership of the object—and the material reality of the object, itself. Here ownership means a belief that baby creates the object in a way that provides a magical sense of control. The experience of control, creation, and ownership is the basis of illusion, spoken of before. This enables a growing sense of confidence in the environment and what is contained within it and of reliability in mother or primary carer and in "mind" or self-experience where omnipotence is felt to be real.

Where the social environment is reliable and attachment is secure, children move more easily from what Fonagy and his colleagues have called "psychic equivalency"—where there is little or no differentiation from mental states and the external environment—to the "pretend phase" in which children from around their third year engage in fantasy play (Fonagy, Gergely, Jurist, & Target, 2004).[46] This fosters development towards a "mentalization phase" in which children grow to have a more finely attuned sense of the mental states—thoughts, feelings, beliefs, desires—of others.

For Winnicott, objects (more properly, concepts) are purely subjective: as experienced in the mind. For Heaton, objects are the world itself as encountered by children's experience of them. Objects are not purely subjective; they also have their own *objective* reality. They have a life of their own. They can disappear or die. They can be lost or taken away. They can behave in ways other than what baby wants or expects. This results in a need for repudiation of the purely subjective in the experience of material objects (and of others). This is a complex process that involves a to-ing and fro-ing between mother and baby and more generally, between baby and world.

The early experience of play promotes a sense of differentiation between the emerging self and the world. There is a movement from undifferentiated (fused) to a separation between what is mine and what is yours, and what is in-between. We can play with those distinctions.

Play in the experience of to-ing and fro-ing between the omnipotent subjectivity of the child's use of objects and their developing conception of them and their independent behaviour (or mother's handling of them) can be immensely exciting. While we might detect a sexual quality in this language, *this process is not sexual.* In an earlier psychoanalytic language, the instincts are not engaged. This is one reason play is developmental for babies and small children, whereas sexual interference, instinctual arousal, exciting their bodies sexually, is counter-developmental. The body is employed in play, but sexual arousal threatens play and risks turning it into something else. On this point, Winnicott is staunch: "in seduction some external agency exploits the child's instincts and helps to annihilate the child's sense of existing as an autonomous unit, making playing impossible" (1971, p. 52). Playing may well be exciting, indeed often is, but this is not the same as sexual excitement. It does not have to be devoid of *eros*[47] but here the sexuality is the child's own and not imposed upon or elicited by someone else.

Play is similarly developmental for adults, for whom sexual excitement is optional. Babies can become absorbed in their own play without direct participation by mother, or anyone. The primary carer can even be forgotten for a time and then remembered. Mother, or carer,

---

[46] This work shares my view that psychology and psychoanalysis have not taken sufficient account of "the developmental processes that underpin the agentive self …" (p. 3) and promotes a developmental reorientation of attachment theory based on interpersonal experience. "Mentalized affectivity" refers to the capacity to connect to the meaning of your emotions (p. 15) in the service of the development of a psychological self. This, in turn, mediates your experience of the world, a position resonant with *Meaning-Fullness*.

[47] The term "eros" has many different usages. Here, I mean "life energy", more specifically it is the underlying energy or quality that is generative of the erotic, and more generally, that which gives pleasure in living.

reflects back what is happening in the play, as needed. Again, play gives a sense of confidence and reliability in the continuity of a caring environment and in children's own ability to lose themselves, thereby being wholly absorbed in the experience of play and of creation/destruction that characterises it. This is generative of the early origins of a capacity to trust in the relationship between a child who plays and a mother or carer who facilitates play; such faith is a basis for living, experiencing space and time in their right order, feeling real and alive, and feeling that living matters, is meaningful.

> Play facilitates emotional growth and health.

Playing must be the child's own in this regard. The imposition of strong direction, order, and rules in the play of children induces compliance and is more likely to produce "good" children than confident and creative ones. Of course, many parents want their children to be *good* without realising the compromise to the child's own development and personality formation. You might be successful in producing a child who never gets into trouble but also never figures out what makes life worth living. When children are allowed, even encouraged, to play on their own terms, there is mess and noise. This might not be comfortable for adults but is developmental for children.

Play is not entirely *inside* the child; it is not a purely mental experience. It is also not something that happens exclusively in the *outside* world. There is an in-between dimension, an intermediate area, a transitional space, where play takes place. We are using metaphors of "space" to describe a type of experience, an activity, and a process. Children become absorbed and preoccupied in this play space to the point that everything else "disappears". Children invest themselves, their feelings, imaginings, energy, and dreams, into play in accord with their creative capacities. In that moment, it matters so much that nothing else matters.

When I complained about the lack of milk in my imaginary tea, though I was playing, I had left the realm of play—for Lucy. She admonished me: USE YOUR IMAGINATION!! and thereby reinserted me back into the realm of her pretend play. If you're drinking imaginary tea, surely you can only add imaginary milk …

> Play is the poetry of childhood experience.

I am not thinking so much of poetry in its structure as metrical verse but the way that poetry takes you beyond yourself. It means something more than its literal expression, a lofty thought expressed beautifully.[48] The poetry of childhood experience resides in the way play takes a child beyond simply being or doing. There is a reaching for *something*, building, dismantling, creating, destroying, imagining, then re-imagining. We could say the same about music; play is the music of childhood experience. Play makes children's experience sing. (It can also make them scream!)

Could play be the poetry of adult experience, too? Play occurs in the service of symbol-formation and ultimately of meaning-making. What does "symbol-formation" mean in this context? Personal symbols refer to what you make of things, what they mean to you and how you connect to them. So, a flag can be a symbol of a country, or I can make a flag that is a symbol of my family, or my estate. My wedding ring is a symbol of my love and commitment to my wife. An anchor is a symbol for my football team. Symbols are informed by meaning and their formation is key to how you assign meaning and value to things, activities, and people. If a soldier gives their life for their country, it is because the symbol of country means that much. It is not child's play when we pledge allegiance to a flag or when a coffin is draped in one.

Meaningful play, play that matters to a child, begins with parenting and with the child's own self and then develops into something that can occur with other children and adults. This leads to group experience and cultural activities. For adults, shared playing is cultural experience. In sharing the experience of a classical music concert with the audience, there is group reverie in the collective delight of the performance. It doesn't have to be highbrow. The same applies to a rock concert—I love both! Nothing makes me feel more Australian than going to an Australian Football League game with my son, dressed in purple—our team's colour—and sharing with 60,000 other people the combined frenzy of excitement, buzz of triumph, and roar of celebratory noise when our team wins. (Occasionally.)

There is a precariousness in play that refers to the ongoing interplay between what goes on in the child's or adult's way of conceptualising what is happening and the perception of what is happening. As I said before, what is precarious is the uncertainty of relating self to world and vice versa and the endeavour to sort out what is what, what you bring to it and what it brings to you. Neither can be pinned down, defined exactly, or determined absolutely—neither is a wholly separable or isolable field.

Winnicott believes that playing is essential in both child and adult development because it is through playing that you develop your capacities to be creative. Indeed, *Playing and Reality* (1971) is regarded as Winnicott's theory of creativity. Self-discovery emerges through play, and specifically through the play of making or finding meaning in the process. Indeed, what "self" *means* is constituted in no small measure by discovering, or creating, what *things* mean to you. In this sense of creativity, self is both discovered and made at once.

---

[48] When Shakespeare was originally performed there was no need for theatrical direction as to how to give emotional expression because it was "built into" the structure of the language. It happened organically in the act of speaking the verse. The play's the thing …

> What it means to be you,
> depends on what is meaningful to you.

One of my children discovered that he liked pottery and indeed had a talent for it. It brought together the earthiness of moulding clay with his hands and artistic elements of designing and glazing the objects he made. In this simple example, you can see how part of his sense of self is realised in this "discovery" which forms an element in a creative process. Creativity refers both to your emerging, evolving sense of self and to what self makes. Is pottery play or work? Could it be both at once?

Play, affective neuroscience, and therapy

Winnicott's views on play are well supported by the work of neuroscientist and psychology professor Jaak Panksepp, who works at the interface between neuroscience and psychoanalysis. The book *The Archaeology of Mind* (Panksepp & Biven, 2012) provides an evidence base for the importance of supportive relationships in general and play specifically for optimal emotional development. Play helps teach both children and animals with whom they can develop cooperative relationships and who to avoid. There are lessons in the dynamics of power, where do you stand in the hierarchy of a range of competitive activities.

> Currently, some of the more boisterous forms of rough-and-tumble play in human children tend to be discouraged by parents. Few of them consider the developmental fact that diminished opportunities for physical play may have undesirable maturational consequences, such as poorly controlled hyperactive urges that can become so severe as to be pathologized, and are all too often given labels such as Attention-Deficit Hyperactivity Disorder (ADHD) (Panksepp, 2007b). (2012, p. 355)

Stimulant medication (typically amphetamine-based) suppresses the impulse to play whereas Panksepp's research shows that abundant daily play reduces ADHD in rats. (Tangentially, rats laugh when tickled and if tickled after being exposed to a fearful situation, the power of the negative affect is diminished (p. 464)). For Panksepp, play is not initially learned. "It is innate. The evidence indicates that PLAY is one of the primary-process, genetically determined social urges" (Panksepp & Biven, 2012, p. 356). He speculates that both play and dreaming

> may help organize information in the brain in ways that promote higher-order affective responses to future life events. In other words, maybe both play and dreaming allow

animals to test solutions to complex problems that they confront in real life. If so, we suspect that playfulness should have a bigger role in psychotherapy than it currently does. (2012, pp. 374–375)

This sentiment echoes Winnicott.

For those interested in brain science, Panksepp cites a recent, comprehensive brain gene-expression analysis that shows about a third of the 1,200 brain genes evaluated in the frontal cortical regions were rapidly modified by play and therefore he assumes "the dynamic brain changes evoked by play facilitate brain growth and maturation, perhaps epigenetically creating prosocial circuits of the brain" (2012, p. 380). The implication here is that play facilitates the creation of new neuronal pathways and helps the development of existing ones through neuroplasticity that supports our capacities for socialisation.

Play takes children to the limit of their emotional knowledge and understanding where they encounter conflicting feelings. Caring adult supervision needs to help children work through these issues. Panksepp concludes: "These considerations highlight the importance of PLAY in the social development of the child" (2012, p. 381). And I would add: promote greater possibilities for mental health as children develop into adults.

> "… children cannot become fully human without play."
> (Panksepp, 2012, p. 387)

The penultimate chapter of *The Archaeology of Mind* considers how play facilities rapid changes in psychotherapy. Panksepp is seeking a synthesis between affective neuroscience and therapy practices. He acknowledges the principal place of the therapeutic relationship and how successful outcomes in therapy depend upon the quality of attachment between patients and clinicians (2012, p. 462). I think Panksepp would like to build a bridge between the more biologically orientated psychiatrists and the more experiential, emotion-focused psychotherapies. Referring to psychiatric diagnosis, he says: "thinking needs to be restructured along the lines of emotional endophenotypes rather than artificial syndromal thinking (Panksepp, 2006a)" (2012, p. 463). This is a different criticism of the DSM from mine in Chapter 2. Endophenotypes refer to the genetic contributions of psychological or behavioural phenomena. He continues:

And many therapists currently recognize that optimal progress will only be achieved if they engage sincerely with patients' emotional dynamics, and to work creatively and sensitively to facilitate the restructuring of patients' affective lives, without neglecting that humans are also fundamentally cognitive beings. So far, the multidimensional therapeutic work remains more of an art than a science. Just as in the skilled playing of a musical instrument, clinicians need solid, rigorous, and practiced techniques, as well as broad-based knowledge of relevant, empirically founded theory, to support flights of inspiration and breakthrough engagements that mark true clinical artistry. (2012, pp. 463–464)

This relates to why I call psychotherapy "an improvisational art".

Panksepp believes that play is as important for adults as for children. "The capacity for emotional resilience is increased by direct physically playful engagements" (2012, p. 464). And lastly:

Any therapist who can capture the therapeutic moment in mutually shared joy episodes will have brought the client to the very doorstep, the wellspring of happy living. To the extent that the patient can remain there, in both body and mind, one may have offered one of the greater emotional gifts that psychotherapy can ever provide. PLAY should have a very special place in psychophysical therapies, from childhood to old age. (2012, pp. 465–466)

CHAPTER 8

Creativity: living falsely or authentically

> *If you think dealing with issues like worthiness and authenticity and*
> *vulnerability are not worthwhile because there are more pressing issues,*
> *like the bottom line or attendance or standardized test scores,*
> *you are sadly, sadly mistaken. It underpins everything.*
>
> Brené Brown

It is creative apperception more than anything else that makes the individual feel that life is worth living. Contrasted with this is a relationship to external reality which is one of compliance, the world and its details being recognized but only as something to be fitted in with or demanding adaptation. Compliance carries with it a sense of futility for the individual and is associated with the idea that nothing matters, and that life is not worth living. (Winnicott, 1971, p. 65)

To know what makes life worth living, consider what prevents it. Winnicott's quote above points to the role of compliance and feelings of futility that follow in its wake. It is not simply being subject to compliance—all of us are to a degree. Abiding by the law, paying taxes, and following the rules of the road are all examples. Excessive compliance creates a mode of being Winnicott called the "false self", involving being "good", doing what is expected and trying to be what (you think) others want you to be. This drives inauthentic behaviours and a feeling of falseness leading to futility.[49]

---

[49] The Winnicottian and the Laingian versions of "false self" are similar.

One patient, Sarah, looked shocked and uneasy when I suggested there was a third possibility other than being either good or bad. She couldn't fathom it. She had spent her life *trying to* be good in the misguided belief that her success would qualify her to be loved. She didn't feel it had worked, not that she felt unloved, but she didn't feel that her mother, in particular, was as emotionally attuned and attentive as she would have liked. Being good was simply what had always been expected.

"What is the third possibility?" Sarah asked me. I said: "Doing what you want." She had no such orientation. She understood "doing what you want" to be selfish. I replied "Such a persecuting judgement becomes a jail-keeper. Following your own desire doesn't have to compromise anyone else."

Our culture is shifting with respect to what it means to be a woman and what it means to be a man, or to be gender non-binary or any other gender. Many patients, especially women, have been raised to accommodate others as their priority, such that the question "What do you want?" doesn't arise. This was the case for Sarah.

Apperception refers to what you make of your perceptions based on past experience and the way your perceptions are affected in the present. You bring something from your past experience to your present experience as you process your experience of the world. What can we understand by putting "apperception" together with "creative" as Winnicott does above: "creative apperception"? Your apperceptions, what you've learned, become formalised as concepts that are held more or less rigidly. There is an interplay between concepts and perceptions. We need to be careful not to let our concepts distort perceptions if what is perceived in the present is different from the past. Otherwise, conceptions become preconceptions even when "things" are not consistent.

The more you suspend preconceptions, a greater sense of freshness arises in your direct experience. This principle is embodied in the current popularity of mindfulness. There will still be a question as to what you make of what you find there, in the interplay, which has important implications for apperception. Suspending preconceptions requires you to know something about your preconceptions, in a sense, to know yourself, know how you operate, mentally and emotionally, know your prejudices. The way to overcome bias in the service of working towards objectivity is to know your biases and suspend them. This takes a measure of creativity brought to your apperceptions—the result is a freedom that allows for genuine choices.

James had been bitten by a dog as a child. It was easy to understand why he was afraid of dogs as an adult. Even the tamest, gentlest dogs made him a little wary. Saying that not all dogs bite people made no difference. He knew that already.

Margot had fallen off her bike as a child and hadn't been back on a bike since. She had been scraped and bruised badly and the fear stayed with her. Her friends kept going away together on cycling trips. They felt exhilarated from the long distances travelled in the day. Then, they had a great deal of fun in the evenings after cycling. She was tired of missing out.

James was quite prepared to forego the ways that a dog can be a best friend because of his one bad experience. Margot didn't mind not having a dog, but she did mind missing out on fun with her friends. She re-learned to cycle safely in a park where no cars were allowed and eventually could get on the road and join her friends. Here, doing what she wanted was the motivating factor that helped Margot overcome her fearful apperception about cycling. We could say fear of cycling gave way to fear of missing out (FOMO) on fun with her friends.

Margot had three former boyfriends; all had cheated on her. It was easy to understand her feeling mistrustful of her fourth, James. It was a clear bias that arose from her past experiences. James was the most trustworthy, faithful guy on the planet and the relationship was undermined by her inability to trust him. *All men cheat*—it's probably just a matter of time. Or do they? James is not "all men". Should she take the risk and trust him while away on a cycling trip or should she trust her past experience?

Knowing your biases and suspending them gives you a choice.

Margot was no longer fearful cycling but being away from James for a week gave her anxiety. He reassured her and did all he could to make her feel safe. But past experience can have a haunting presence.

If you can, meet present experience with a fresh attitude, an openness, and a suspension of preconceptions and prejudices. Yet, you are naive if you don't learn from past experience. Don't forget everything you have ever been through. Only fools fail to learn lessons, they are condemned to repeat painful experiences, and they recur with uncanny regularity. Somewhere there is a happy medium where apperceptions are not hardened into concrete and your memories are still available as a resource from which to draw when needed. Finding that happy medium is what I mean in this context by creative.

Prejudice destroys the freshness of the present.
Thus it kills time.

Past emotional injuries and traumas can inform prejudices and preconceptions that then become projected upon your view of the future, a perpetual treadmill of anxious apprehension and re-enactment.

"Creative apperception *more than anything else* makes us feel that life is worth living" (Winnicott, 1971, p. 65, my emphasis). The happy medium involves learning from past experience, remembering what's gone before, but also recognising that present experience is not necessarily the same. The creativity brought to the present requires you to be present, to be sentient, alive to what is happening now and alert to the differences from everything that has gone before. Life *feels* worth living when you are fully in it and of it in a creative relation that is generative of meaning, as time unfolds. You must give as you are given-to.

Many patients, in my experience, have lived through and survived the nightmare of their childhood (or some portion of it) only to feel unsafe, terribly vulnerable, suspicious, and vigilant in a present situation that offers a loving, caring, safe and secure environment and relationships—if only they can believe it. Creative apperception recognises this difference and embraces it, thereby validating faith.

* * *

To recap: excessive or compulsive compliance is the basis of the false self and prevents the creativity that needs to be brought to your apperceptions. Falseness arises out of having to fit in, do what is expected, look to others for indications as to who you are and how you should be. The source of your sense of yourself is others or, more accurately, your own way of looking to others for such indications. You are interpreting what others want or expect. This is one meaning of self-consciousness: what you think others think of you. There is a high degree of adaptation to be or do what (you think) you are supposed to.

What if no one is actually requiring anything? Where is the self in this? Where is your authenticity? Where is a place for original thought or genuine feelings? Where is your spontaneity, the organic productions that flow from yourself as true expressions of who you are, how you feel, what you want, and where you're going—without undue regard for anyone else's opinion or critical judgement? That is what authenticity means in practice.

Of course, if you are taking a course of study, there are requirements with which you must comply. If you are in a relationship, then there are agreements and conditions to comply with, as I say in *How Two Love* (Resnick, 2016) and if you are employed, then you have an employment contract that sets out requirements to be complied with. And so on. This is not false; it is necessary and can be a positive choice. There are rules of conduct whether you recognise them or not, whether explicit or not. The penalties for non-compliance can be severe, the consequences compromising. This is not false either. It is when compliance is a basis for living, however, that futility grows to dominate how you feel. Everything is pre-determined, so there is no space for creative input or output. No two-way traffic. Therefore, nothing much matters. Hence, it is only a short hop to feeling Imposter Syndrome or, worse: that life is not worth living. I have one client after another who feels like that, more or less.

> Compulsive compliance makes living feel futile.

When people feel this way and commence psychotherapy, an opportunity to play, as a key part of the process, presents itself—that is, assuming the style of therapy is open and not already pre-determined. *Oh no! Another questionnaire—now I have to comply with that!*

If patients have to comply with what professionals require of them, how will anyone ever overcome falseness? And how will their answers to questions be anything other than false, based on what they think is expected of them? You want to be seen in a particular light. You don't want to be thought badly of. Now, you are anticipating what the assessor will make of your answers and so adjust them accordingly. Then, you pretend to agree with the result. Perhaps I have a preconception and prejudice against questionnaires (I definitely do). I know some are written to throw patients off and counter the tendency of patients to give answers they think are expected. The writers believe they can overcome this issue with clever tricks and asking similar questions in different ways. This just seems like a ludicrous game to me, where the questioner is trying to anticipate the patient's responses and the patient is trying to anticipate what the assessor is anticipating.

Psychotherapy works best when therapists can suspend their preconceptions, not make undue demands, and meet their patients with a fresh and open attitude, to discover this unique person coming to consult—every session. Who knows? Maybe they will even discover themselves.

Judgements are part of the natural flow of consciousness, they can be thought without being made.

> If mental health practices operate through a false self structure, they contribute to futility, rather than to overcoming it.

Here is a brief example:

> A client of mine in therapy felt unhappy that she was still suffering from intrusive thoughts. What if something happens? What if this red colour on a website means the devil is involved? What if I do something I shouldn't? If I find a woman attractive, do you think it means I'm gay? Her doctor referred her to a psychologist who, following

CBT, suggested my client practise "postponement". Whenever you have an intrusive thought, just tell yourself you'll worry about that later. Six sessions and she was done.

My client did practice postponement and felt happy that it worked, albeit only temporarily.

This account will be added to psychology's evidence base of successes as it helped her to avoid her thoughts and feelings and she was pleased with the result.[50] Should this be regarded as evidence of efficacy though? My client complied with what she was told to do. Her relief from intrusive thoughts lasted two weeks. Then she forgot about postponement. If anything, she seemed to harbour a renewed sense of urgency as to why the thoughts kept recurring and what they meant. She told me that postponement had made her feel more futile about resolving this issue because it was being avoided. It was as if the subtext of the suggestion to practise postponement was. "We can't help you because no one really knows what to do to stop intrusive thoughts. That's why you should put it off and worry about it later. If you keep putting it off, you will never have to deal with it. It will just go away."

But it didn't.[51]

Creative play

Creative play can refer to practically anything. In therapy, a patient can find an interesting way to tell the story of something that happened to them or fantasise about their wildest dreams or tease me about looking tired. Outside of therapy, creative play can occur through

- a beautifully cooked meal expressing love
- a new hair style or a new suit of clothes
- cleaning the car or fitting an accessory
- the production of an artwork, sculpture, poem, or piece of writing
- a musical composition
- a joke
- a song or a riff on the guitar
- a different way of applying make-up
- an architect's inspiration in design
- growing vegetables or flowers

---

[50] As my client was quite happy with this result, I didn't say a negative word about it. In professional practice, it is important for clients to have their own experiences and form their own opinions—as I'm espousing here—without being undermined, as happens all too often between competing professionals. I admit I was squirming inside. I work to help people face things and develop capacities to cope with what is painful and difficult, rather than to develop better strategies of avoidance.

[51] Two further years of psychotherapy sessions later, this client declared she'd had no further intrusive thoughts, and so didn't refer to them again. There was no technique applied.

- an innovation in business
- breaking into a dance move when a song comes on the radio
- a different way to trade shares or cryptocurrencies
- a scientific research project, or
- a new product to sell.

There are an infinite number of possibilities; it depends on how you go about it. Does the artwork come from a place deep within yourself or is it something you think your mentor would approve of? Is the creation an expression of self or of an internalised parent or teacher? Is cooking dinner for your family part of the domestic slog of everyday living, an obligation, or an opportunity to express love through creative possibilities of providing nutriment and sensual pleasure in eating? Is making it enjoyable or burdensome? Can you see the difference between authentic creativity and false-self productions? This is what makes the difference between feeling fulfilled or feeling empty. It also makes the difference between other peoples' enjoyment of what you make or a feeling of guilty indebtedness for your suffering.

I do not expect you to dance through life feeling joy and singing "Kumbaya" all the way. I am raising questions for your consideration: look at how you feel doing the everyday tasks that constitute your way of living. Are you happy doing what you're doing? Does it feel right to be responsible for those tasks? Purposeful? Satisfying? Rewarding? Are you doing what you most want to be doing and are you happy-enough doing it? Or not? What are you saying as you execute your tasks—"I love you and it feels good to give as an expression of that" or "I wish I didn't have to do this every day, the tedium is killing me, I feel wretched and hard-done-by, poor me"? Are you a victim of circumstance rueing your lot in life or choosing positively to make something out of your position in the scheme of things? Most activities can be done either like a robot or from the heart.[52]

Some forms of creativity aim to create a self, as if the creator needs the product to make the self emerge as an identity. This is unlikely to be rewarding if the endeavour is to relieve oneself of an underlying emptiness. It takes the form of a search for recognition rather than suspending ego gratification in the service of giving birth to something with its own identity, something that can be set free to live its own life. Then, people can have a relationship to the product independently of its creator.

> Henry was a retired university professor who was writing a book. Although he had consulted me for depression, we spent most of the time in sessions talking about his book. It became clear that his ultimate aim for the book was for him to be loved, admired, and recognised for his knowledge and brilliance. I had no doubt that he was knowledgeable,

---

[52] The story of *The Stepford Wives* (1975) comes to mind here. The men of Stepford did not want authentic, spirited women with personalities of their own and so turned them into smiling servile robots.

and I could see his brilliance. That is not what I said, however: "No one cares about you. Your readers are primarily interested in what you can do for them."

It sounded harsh and I admit Henry looked taken aback when I said this. He came back the following week and said: "I thought a lot about what you said last week. I felt hurt at first but then to my surprise I felt my depression lifting. I felt freed up to apply myself to the book which I did while I hadn't really been able to get down to it before. It was kind of liberating."

He had harboured a fantasy that his imaginary readers would celebrate him because of his (imagined) work. Later, he realised that he had lived much of his life in the futile attempt to gain others' approval, admiration, and love. I said he was more likely to write a successful book if he could express what he had to say without seeking positive affirmation as the main driver of the work.

Often, the need to avoid disapproval or, worse, censure, reproach, criticism, or, worst of all, the cruel, cold, silent indifference of being ignored as if you didn't exist—can be indicators of a false self. Put the other way around, the drive to elicit attention and approval, and more specifically, praise, affirmation, recognition, love, and admiration are all further indicators of false-self being, at least in part. There is a hunger for narcissistic supply. When Henry put that aside, he was freed up to play with his own ideas and see what he could make of them. He started to enjoy the writing process. It felt creative, whereas previously it had been a grind, or he was bogged down, and that fuelled his depression.

It's not that we should be completely immune to the effects of negative or positive feedback. It becomes questionable when we are overly driven by a need to elicit the positive or avoid the negative. We can recognise these features in the behaviour of children because they are part of the process of growing up. As adults, many fear if they are not what others want, demand, or expect, then they will not be accepted at all.

Henry's psychology can also be understood in terms of attachment theory referenced here as it has become one of the dominant theories informing early child development and now applied to adults as well. John Bowlby, the English psychiatrist, psychoanalyst, and psychologist, pioneered attachment theory. He was greatly influenced by Winnicott though their respective approaches to child development took different paths. Generally, psychoanalysts did not embrace Bowlby's work at the time. Much of his research was based on ethology (the study of animal behaviour) rather than Freudian ideas. And Bowlby argued that children were responding to real-life events, not to the unconscious fantasies that were close to the hearts and minds of his psychoanalytic supervisors (Melanie Klein and others). Despite these differences, Bowlby's work and its further development into empirically testable and verifiable ideas (especially by the Developmental Psychologist Mary Ainsworth) has gained credence amongst those involved with child and adult emotional development.[53]

---

[53] During my professional training at the Philadelphia Association in London in the late 1970s, R. D. Laing showed trainees the film made by John Bowlby and James Robertson called *A Two-Year-Old Goes to Hospital* (1952)

Of relevance here is that Bowlby believed that much of mental disorder in adults can be understood as arising from developmental issues of childhood, as I am espousing in this book. Despite their earlier *attachment* to classical theories of unconscious fantasy, now psychoanalysts, along with most contemporary psychiatrists and paediatricians, have embraced the ideas of attachment theory.

Briefly, for Bowlby "attachment" refers to the affectionate ties babies show for their carers. The attachment relationship grows out of a need for safety (and comfort) and—of great importance—is reciprocal between adults and children. As such, it is a relational theory. Attachment is said to develop in phases:

- Asocial—first six weeks of infancy
- Indiscriminate attachment—six weeks to seven months
- Specific attachment—seven to nine months on
- Multiple attachments—eighteen months on.

And attachment styles develop as different types:

- Secure
- Resistant (also called anxious-ambivalent)
- Avoidant (also called anxious-avoidant)
- Disorganised.

The above can be equated with degrees of developmental difficulty (descending = greater difficulty) correlating with more severe issues in adult relationships and self-esteem.

The text cited previously by Fonagy and his colleagues, *Affect Regulation, Mentalization, and the Development of the Self* (2004), is envisaged by the authors as a further development and reformulation of Bowlby's attachment theory.

Let's return to Henry. He had been writing his book and, in a more general way, had lived his life doing things for other people with the aim of eliciting their love and appreciation. In the early days of attachment theory, this was called "cupboard love", especially in Britain. Henry was fundamentally insecure in his attachment to his significant others and, in his own mind, he had to write a brilliant book to secure his position in his relationships, a false-self approach. Then, he found himself bogged down and unable to get on with it and grew depressed. I startled him with my comment about others not caring about him and only wanting what he could offer them. Confronting his attachment pattern in this way seemed to jolt him out of it, at least in that moment, such that he felt better and could get on with his work *for its own sake*. The point I was making, in different words was:

---

showing a young child affected by brief separation from their primary caregiver. I was moved by the suffering and visible effects of loss and especially the damage upon the bond with the primary carer, the mother. It sensitised me to the impact of separation, and I never forgot it.

> Give for its own sake and for the benefit of others, not just for what you can get in return.[54]

In the conceptual framework of mentalization, if Henry could read the minds of others—desiring to receive what they could from his work, as I indicated—he would be less preoccupied with being loved or admired, more focused on what he could offer, and correspondingly less depressed and more engaged in the writing. This was the case for a while, a theme we return to as we go, in ongoing therapy.

False self, decompensation, breakdown

Some people develop false selves primarily as a survival strategy. Others are more concerned to position themselves in the best possible light. Whatever the motivation, the transition from growing up to grown-up is also a transition from false-self being to authentic being. This is where developmental psychotherapy comes in, when needed.

Other features of the false self include copying and imitating. In its more extreme form this can include plagiarising and stealing. It is perhaps a specialised form of stealing in the service of being-like or trying to become the person who is stolen from.

> Many years ago, a patient in psychotherapy began consulting me for a depressed, empty sort of feeling. The next thing I knew he was growing a beard and trimming it exactly like mine. Then he bought a pair of shoes identical to mine. He started dressing in a way that resembled my style of clothes, quite different from how he had first looked. At that time, I smoked cigars. I don't even know how he discovered this because I never smoked while working. But he announced that he had developed a taste for cigars. Then he started talking about buying a blue car—like mine! They say imitation is a form of flattery, but I found this alarming and not at all flattering. In fact, the more he carried on like that, the more unwell he seemed. The more he became like me, the more I found him disagreeable (funny, that).
>
> It felt like he was desperately searching for a self of his own and needed to take something of mine for himself. The more he looked and acted like me (he began using certain phrases and idioms of speech he got from me and gesticulated with his hands as I do—it began to feel like looking into a mirror) the more he seemed like a false self. I tried to

---

[54] This point can be related to the previous discussion of the difference between praxis-for-its-own-sake and productivity. There is also giving for its own sake and giving to produce a desired outcome.

point this out to him, rather gently. He denied that it had any significance. He liked my shoes, so why shouldn't he buy the same ones? He had been thinking of growing a beard for some time. Lots of people smoke cigars and drive blue cars, like mine.

Some people only seem to bring their false selves into therapy. We can do an entire course of long-term therapy over five years or more and never reach beyond the false self. Then, clients invariably leave having a good understanding of things, able to explain why they are as they are, but do not feel entirely "real" underneath that. The crucial challenge for therapy is to get through layers of falsely constructed self-experience and behaviour to the core of an underlying disturbance. This can be frightening, as what is underneath can be a somewhat traumatised, under-developed person who feels like nothing, not even a person at all.

There is a risk of decompensation. Decompensation is a psychiatric term for being unable to function because an underlying condition is dominating. Former defences are not strong enough to compensate, or are falling away, necessarily. Falling apart, going to pieces, disintegrating can be expressions of decompensation. This kind of fragmentation and breakdown can be truly alarming and there is a risk of the person's not being able to function independently at all. When a client is an adult who holds responsibility for small children, a business, a professional practice, or a multi-national corporation, then this is deeply worrying and holds potential consequences that ripple out to affect others. Yet, breakdown is sometimes necessary to attend to the core of a deep disturbance that has been buried and hidden for years, even decades. Ideally, therapists negotiate the need to uncover and treat deep disturbance and minimise decompensation at the same time. This is a tricky balance that requires skill and sensitivity. There is no volume control to reduce the intensity of disturbance when breakdown occurs. Unfortunately, I find fewer therapists are being trained to work with deep underlying disturbance or psychotic conditions. It is the "too-hard basket".[55]

Not every person with a false self has such extreme underlying disturbance. The false self involves a defensive strategy, a personality organisation that keeps things at a distance, keeps them from mattering too much, and protects vulnerability. It avoids conflict and confrontation. It veers away from anger and rage. It diminishes susceptibility to depression, despondency, dysphoria, and low moods. Sometimes, the false self is accompanied by a manic defence or hypomania. The manic defence refers to an elevated mood that denies the gravity of things, deflects emotional suffering, and can take the form of being animated, hyper, revved, energetic, dynamic, and humourous, entertaining, cheeky, full of laughs. The hypomanic character can be convincing, can go into a meeting with his bank manager and convince them to lend hundreds of thousands of dollars to fund a business that involves buying washing machines on the certainty they can be sold for massive profits. Such schemes are rarely thought through, are

---

[55] Addressing the Royal College of Psychiatrists in Ireland, R. D. Laing famously said "The reason people are locked away in mental institutions is not because they are suffering, but because they are insufferable!"

unrealistic, and almost never succeed. Yet, the hypomanic person might get the loan whereas the sober businessperson with a solid proposal might not. This is just one example.

Hypomanic defences can exist separately from false-self organisation. Part of the false-self function is to prevent the person from realising their own false-self organisation. Often, underneath it, there is a relatively unformed personality. People don't know how they *really* feel or what they think about things. Their orientation has been directed away from their own true desire, emotion, or position about things, and focused more towards others. Others become the primary reference point for how to be. It is as if the false-self person had a radar dish circling to pick up others' desires, what others think of them, want of them, expect of them, demand of them (or think they know). It is as if their value as a person is based wholly on accommodating others in this way. It is as if their value as a person doesn't count *unless* they are of value to others *on their terms*. The false-self person often does not have much of a sense of entitlement, ownership, or rights to make demands upon others or protest mistreatment. It is a particularly difficult position for parents, leaving them ineffectual and lacking in authority. Kids can sense it.

As before, there is no defined field that can separate out authentic and false absolutely. These are qualities, tendencies, or trends that come to the fore in one moment or recede in another. Some people function as false selves all the time while others do some of the time but not always. If you are not a false-self person but choose to be compliant, acquiescent, or accommodating, then that is a positive, authentic choice. It is possible to be false in one relationship and authentic in another. You might wish to be diplomatic in one situation and confronting in another. Being compliant without question or choice is what I mean by false-self functioning.

Impingements

False-self functioning can arise from the experience of impingements in early childhood and then it re-creates the conditions for further impingements in your adult life. I suggest looking at your own experience for a moment. Practically everyone contends with some impingements. Consider for a moment: do you ever feel like you lurch from one impingement to the next and that life consists primarily of a series of events that make demands upon you, require your attention, money, and emotional response, and that there is little in it for you? You might rather not even be doing it, if only you could get out of it. Here is the worst example I know.

> Jordan woke to a phone call from a friend whose car had broken down. The friend had to be in court and needed help. Jordan jumped in his own car, met his friend, and took him to court. Then Jordan offered to get his friend's car towed so it was not left in a bad position on the side of the road. The towing company indicated it would be there within the hour but two hours later, they had not appeared. Jordan got a parking ticket

because he didn't want to leave his friend's car unattended for fear of missing the tow truck. Finally, the tow truck did appear but had to be paid at the time. Jordan paid, even though his friend had not agreed to the cost. In fact, his friend was unhappy later upon hearing how high the charge was. Jordan felt off-side with his friend *because he helped him out*. He was out of pocket on the tow truck and the parking fine. (He could hardly ask his friend to cover the fine).

It gets worse.

From there, Jordan went to work. He was not late, but he was soiled from dealing with the broken-down car. This is not acceptable for working in a restaurant. His boss was unhappy with him. Jordan was waiting on tables in a sour mood. The customers registered this and complained to him: "You look like you got out of bed on the wrong side this morning." He was pissed off, irritable, and annoyed that everything seemed so difficult. In this state, he slipped, bumped into the sharp corner of a sideboard, fell, and dropped a tray of main courses. The food was wasted and had to be replaced, the customers were angry for having to wait, the kitchen staff were angry for having to replace the meals.

It gets worse.

Meanwhile, Jordan hurt his back with the fall. He needed to see a physical therapist. The only appointment he could get was Saturday afternoon, but he and his girlfriend had agreed to watch the football game together then, at the pub, on the big screen. She was aggrieved with him because he had to break that date, which she had been looking forward to.

It gets much worse.

After his physio appointment, he drove home, exhausted, and emotionally drained. Someone cut in front of him narrowly missing his front bumper. If he hadn't slammed on the brakes, he would have made contact with that car. He leaned on the horn and, feeling enraged, shouted. The car in front was offended by this honking and swearing which was audible through the open window. The other driver forced him to pull over. He got out of his car, swaggered over, wearing a motorcycle club leather jacket, covered in tattoos and piercings, with an expression on his face that said: "Killing you would give me joy." Jordan wondered if he had a gun.

He threatened to punch Jordan in the face if he had a problem with his driving. Jordan's heart was pounding, his pulse was racing, sweat formed on his brow—he was just about to cop one in the face—when he broke down in tears. It was all too much; he was overwhelmed. The other driver mocked him and left.

Remember: no matter how bad things are—it can always get worse.

Jordan was a wreck by the time he got home, despondent, and self-pitying. He turned on the television, but the internet was down. Practically suicidal, he went to the fridge to grab a beer, his last solace, but alas, his flat-mate was desperate and had finished them off an hour earlier. The note said: "Don't worry, I'll buy some more tomorrow."

What a day! It is a catalogue of impingements, one after another. Although extreme, I have heard countless accounts from clients of this sort of experience. In this account, it seemed like it had little or nothing to do with Jordan. He did the best he could for his friend, for his work, and even by trying to drive safely, but to no avail. It feels like the world is conspiring against him, nothing goes his way. It is hard to see what Jordan did to organise this series of misfortunes, but he is the common denominator. Even though it can be hard to avoid impingements, it must have something to do with him. There is what the world throws at you, too, just when you least expect it—or deserve it!

If your life keeps going like this, with regular impingements, it won't take long before you question why bother. Is it worth living? Many people feel trapped in a pattern like this. *Stop the world, I want to get off.* What can be done about it?

It is a feature of false-self organisation, and the sooner it is addressed, redressed, and, ideally, dismantled in favour of a more authentic way of being, the sooner such impingements stop recurring, or at least diminish. Changing this pattern makes everything feel different even if some impingements happen to everyone. You may not be able to change the world, but something probably does need to change in yourself. You gain a greater sense of agency and make choices that work more in your favour. Relinquishing the false-self way of being reduces the corresponding feelings of futility, frustration, regret, wastefulness, and grief that go with it. Authentic living has a completely different quality. For one thing, it becomes easier to say "no" and for another, to know the difference between "Yes, I can do that for you" and "NO!"

How does a false-self organisation come about in the first place? For Winnicott, when infants adjust their needs unduly to the needs of carers or those upon whom the infant is dependent, a movement towards compliance is initiated. If there is emotional withdrawal or neglect or, alternatively, the primary (especially) carer imposes their needs upon the infant, then the infant's experience will become increasingly characterised as a series of reactions to these impingements. The infant's experience is intruded upon or rejected or possibly abandoned and hence the infant's sense of initiative and spontaneity becomes replaced by a growing sense of futility and despair. There is a corresponding substitution of a false self for the true self, with which I associate the term "authentic self". The need for a defensive organisation such as "the false self" occurs when the child's continuity of being is disrupted by lack of adequate and sufficient care, Winnicott's "good-enough mothering". Then, spontaneity, originality, and creative impulses are diminished or impaired, leaving children to grow up feeling empty, fraudulent, or lacking as a person. Self-doubt informs the foreground of experience and taints self-reflection accordingly. As such, the corresponding apperceptions of experience are projected forward to adult experience as inauthentic. This makes creative apperception harder to reach to, and with that, the feeling that life is worth living or put differently, that "I" am worthwhile.

Winnicott says impingements make it difficult for children to develop into a "true self" or as an authentic individual.

The "individual" then develops as an extension of the shell rather than of the core, and as an extension of the impinging environment. What there is left of a core is hidden away and is difficult to find even in the more far-reaching analysis. The individual then *exists by not being found*. The true self is hidden, and what we have to deal with clinically is the complex *false self* whose function is to keep this true self hidden. (1958, p. 212, original emphasis)

Authenticity brings with it a feeling of acceptance of both the capacities and limitations of the person you are. Further development is desirable and requires work. There tends to be a capacity to think of and care for others that is free from excessive worry of how you are seen by others. Humility is possible without self-degradation.

Authenticity has a quality of care that informs an attitude of doing what you can for others, not more, not less—while understanding the limits of your position. For authentic living to work, care needs to be balanced. No one can prescribe how much care is the right amount, but some people care too much, and others don't care enough. What is this judgement based on? There is no objective scale or measure of how much care is the right amount.

In psychotherapy, caring too much brings intense suffering and creates a feeling in others of your over-investment. What makes it "over-investment" is the sense of going too far, beyond your reach, beyond what is possible. Omnipotence is implied. Some people care about some things more than others. Some people care so much that they are in constant pain over one issue after another: famine, poverty, climate change, war, displaced people, homelessness, child abuse, racism, sexism, homophobia—all are important, of course. I think the segregation of wealth into fewer "hands" is a crime against the great majority of people. What can be done about it?

Perhaps we don't care enough? Caring too much leaves you weakened, if not disabled, whereas not caring at all leaves you lacking in compassion and humanity. Authenticity is informed by care in its right proportion, including for yourself.

Have we arrived at an understanding of Winnicott's statement that "It is creative apperception more than anything else that makes the individual feel that life is worth living" (1971, p. 65)? Early on in this book, we spoke of the existential vacuum, feelings of emptiness, meaninglessness, and purposelessness. Here, our discussion turns to how the false-self way of being generates feelings of futility and the sense that life is not worth living. This is why an experience of psychotherapy needs to be developmental and work towards authenticity. Otherwise, you may be condemned—through no fault of your own—to applying yourself towards compliance, acquiescence, adaptation, fitting in, doing what's expected, and self-consciously avoiding criticism, censure, or disapproval. Creative apperception means you bring something of yourself to the world as you experience it, and receive something from the world, making of it what you will, owning that, and then living out your choices and decisions—independently of what anyone else says or thinks. Such developmental work is a journey towards meaningfullness and a sense of freedom that goes with it.

Masochism and surrender

In one of my favourite articles in the literature from the relational psychoanalysis and psychotherapy group, and one that touches on many of the themes in this book, I turn to Emmanuel Ghent's seminal article distinguishing masochism from surrender.

Ghent paints a vivid picture of the sorts of distortions that occur as a consequence of false-self functioning. A person wanting to be recognised, discovered, or uncovered may also feel defeated once they have registered their own distortions and feel terrified to be seen by others. Rather than defeat, Ghent argues for a more Eastern understanding of surrender, that of transcendence and liberation (1990, p. 216). As described above, the defensive organisation called false self arises out of necessity, usually as a survival strategy. Giving it up—surrender—is no easy task, and perversions of surrender can amount to submission and masochism. Masochism is a term for self-defeat and self-sabotage, and Western thinkers have often wrongly equated that with surrender.

The overcoming of the masochistic tendency involves letting others in, allowing yourself to be known, recognised, and understood without undue fear of psychological annihilation. It involves coming out of hiding—*come out and play*.

Emptiness, dread, and futility are consequences of the false-self position, as are attracting impingements and the sort of dominating dynamics that incur submission. There can be a corresponding depletion of energy, a lifeless or dead feeling, or stuckness. This occurs so commonly in contemporary culture that therapists hear about such experiences on a regular basis. However, the alternative, standing up for oneself, setting boundaries, resisting mistreatment, spontaneous expressions of desire or creativity, freedom from self-consciousness, and the (imagined or real) persecuting judgements of others, and a feeling of vitality—all seem like an elusive dream. This is also why an analysis or therapy that understands and works sensitively with these tendencies is essential for further development of an authentic or true self.[56]

What is at stake here is the very emergence of a sense of self that feels real and holds opportunities for creative experiencing. This notion of development involves making a transition from object relating to object use (discussed more fully in the next chapter) and destroying the projections and misconceptions of others along the way in the service of a more confident sense of externality and difference. As Ghent puts it:

> The essence of both transitional experiencing and the transition into object usage is the heady and wonderful world of creative experiencing wherein self and other have the opportunity to become real. Failures in either or both of these developmental currents leads to the development of one or other variety of false self; from the baby's point of view they might well be called failures of faith. (1990, p. 227)

---

[56] A qualification: true and false self are not an absolute dichotomy or polar opposites, rather these descriptors refer to tendencies across a range of experience and are not identifications set in concrete.

Such failures can come about by impingements from caregivers to the point that a baby or small child will seek further impingements *in order to exist*—or have the feeling of being real in their own right. And this can carry on into adult life, and through distortions or perversions it can become the submissive, masochistic, self-sabotaging tendency. This can be an attempt

> to reengage that area of transitional experiencing, the miscarriage of which impulse or longing appears as masochism or submission. (1990, p. 227)

Some patients find they need affirmation from others not only as admiration for what they've done but more to support the feeling they actually exist at all. In this regard, one of Ghent's patients came upon the word "beinglessness"—a poignant descriptor. He felt a horror of this state but also realised he was drawn to revisit it. Ghent suggests to him:

> by reaching into the is-ness of the circumstances that led to that horror, or the events that did not happen that might have otherwise brought him into being, he is unconsciously seeking a chance to come solidly into being. As the session in question came to a close the patient said, "I have to hold onto this place and never forget it. If I lose it would be like the most important page of a book torn out. The book would be meaningless". (1990, p. 232)

Ontology—the study of being—is at the core of possibilities for meaning-making and of the realisation of a sense of self that feels genuine and alive, overcoming the existential vacuum and the false-self tendency so closely related to it. In the next chapter, we will see how the developmental transition from object relating (that is mental activity) to object use (practical activity) involves surrender in the transcendental sense and involves taking a risk for both the small child and caregiver, and later for the adult patient and therapist.

CHAPTER 9

The object of desire and how to destroy it

There is an invisible strength within us;
when it recognises two opposing objects
of desire, it grows stronger.
Rumi

The opposing objects of which Rumi speaks are the Devil and the Angelic Spirit; they awaken us to the power of choice. How do they?—only if you feel the pull of Evil or the Good, in another language. We grow stronger by exercising choice in our actions, as the forces of opposing influences compel our desires. Strength grows through wrestling with such forces in ourselves if we are awakened by the power of choice.

Notice the profound quality of abstraction in "objects" such as the Devil and Angelic Spirit. Maybe you have your own experience of such objects but to me, they are conceptual and remain as constructions of mind even when "they" are thought to work upon your actions and corresponding consequences and benefits. This chapter is about the way we move from abstraction to action and how destroying the objects of mind clears a path for the movement of choice and the development of mental health.

Object relating and object use

A Winnicottian distinction can be made between object relating and object use. Object relating refers to your idea of things, what they mean to you. For example, writing this book is important to me—I desire it—and is an example of object relating in so far as it requires imagining it, having a vision, working, and playing with thoughts. Object relating is my way of relating to the idea I have of this book. The act of actually writing the text and producing a manuscript and ultimately, a physical book, is an example of object use. Once written, the book holds an independent, separate existence from me and could mean something to others, different from what it means to me, or how I intend it. What goes on "in my head",[57] my thoughts, cannot mean anything to anyone other than myself until they are symbolised, formulated, and written, and so able to be shared.

Object use refers to the materialisation of those thoughts or any other purely mental process such as fantasy, dreams, visions, imaginings, intuitions, or premonitions. Object use has possibilities for sharing with others such that thoughts can become meaningful other than to oneself. An example of the movement from object relating to object use is speaking. Another example: an architect conceives a design for an amazing building, but it cannot hold value for anyone else until it is built, or at very least, drawn.

If you desire a new or different sort of relationship, you could find yourself fantasising about meeting the right partner for a relationship: Mr Right, Ms Ideal, or the Ultimate Non-Binary—this is object relating—the idea of the One. The actual person you get involved with cannot be the ideal object of your mental design—this involves object use, the personal engagement with an actual other person, *this* relationship.

The transition from object relating to object use, from your conception of an object to the manifestation of it, something that can be perceived, involves transitional phenomena. I began to have thoughts of wanting to write a book around 1976. My first book was published in 2016, some forty years later. We could say the process of transitional experiencing covered that time frame and still goes on to this day. Perhaps the forty years was the necessary developmental process to build a capacity that enabled turning thoughts into a book, to see it through.[58]

Winnicott is concerned with the detail of the transitional phenomena from object relating to object usage. Creative doing requires effort but can feel rewarding, if not pleasurable, whereas object relating remains in the closed circuit of your own thoughts. Sometimes, it involves hard thinking, which is exhausting. Object use can have different qualities such as work or play or playful work unless informed by a compulsive drive, in which case it feels more like being oppressed by a tyrant forcing the effort.

> To use an object the subject must have developed a *capacity* to use objects. (Winnicott, 1971, p. 89, original emphasis)

---

[57] This expression is commonly used but there is much written to suggest that thinking does not "go on in our heads", at least not exclusively, even if it might feel like that. Obviously, we do need a functional brain to think.
[58] "Seeing it through" is really saying something: that first book, *How Two Love*, saw thirty iterations of the complete manuscript; I even had it typeset in 2014 but was then told *you can't publish that*! And then a further two years of re-writing before it was good enough to be released.

Transitional experience is one answer to the question of how the capacity to use objects in a creative way develops. Building capacities is also the nature of the therapeutic work of a developmental psychotherapy. There are important implications for how to apply these ideas to adult experiences (as I will show in the long case of Luke in Part IV). People find that being absorbed in creative endeavours helps to lift low moods by shifting from mental activity to physical engagement with the world, by virtue of a practical activity.

The transition from object relating to object use is also a transition from the omnipotent formation of illusion to creative living that is both purposeful and rewarding. It involves a movement from grandiose fantasies of what could be achieved to the ordinary productions of what is possible within the limits of your abilities. (Remember the example of Calvin in Chapter 6.)

Developmentally, it is desirable, relieving, and rewarding to move from object relating to object use.

Get out your mind and into the world.

Of course, this refers to what is creative and beneficial and not what is harmful and destructive. If destructive, then it's preferable to get it out of your thoughts without subjecting the world to it. The world is already suffering from a cumulative history of destructiveness. The developmental leap of destroying mental objects is, itself, an overcoming of the need to destroy external objects, especially each other! For Winnicott, this is the most difficult "thing" in human development:

> In the sequence, one can say that first there is object-relating, then in the end there is object-use; in between, however, is the most difficult thing, perhaps, in human development; or the most irksome of all the early failures that come for mending. This thing that there is in between relating and use is the subject's placing of the object outside the area of the subject's omnipotent control; that is, the subject's perception of the object as an external phenomenon, not as a projective entity, in fact recognition of it as an entity in its own right. (1971, p. 89)

Winnicott is saying something important about recognising the separate and independent existence of things and other people. By "come for mending" he is referring to coming to psychotherapy. The idea of mending suggests something is broken.

This "most difficult thing" is removing your projections. Your projections express what you want this object to be and your sense of control over it. "In its own right" means it is not yours, you don't possess it or them (if a person). Often, it is a part or aspect of yourself that is projected. In this context, object means external object. What makes it difficult is that external objects are always the objects of your perception. How you see something is affected by your perspective: *your way of seeing* and what you make of it (apperception), your idea of that external object. What you make of what you see can alter (your conception of) the object and what it means to you. Are they one and the same? For perception to be free from preconceptions, perception must precede apperception through a pre-reflective attitude. *Are you seeing it as it is, in itself, or are you seeing what you put there?* The difficulty is knowing the difference. An example helps to see how this works and what makes it difficult.

> One patient, Max, was convinced his girlfriend, Sam, had been cheating. He accused her again and again. She was distraught; nothing she could say or do would convince him otherwise. He accused her of cheating with both other men and women. Sam claimed to be "as straight as an arrow". Her friendship group all supported her protestations of innocence.
>
> Of course, we never know with absolute certainty, but all the evidence suggested that Max was projecting. He had paid for sex when he and Sam were on a break. His accusations were so persistent, unyielding, and certain that most people regarded him as delusional, probably just another example of male coercive control.

I had sessions with Max, who was desperate to be believed. I had some sessions with Sam, too, and she was convincing. And I had sessions with both together where they fought it out. So, when I say the most difficult thing is to identify your projections and remove them, this becomes a tricky example. It can be impossible to know whether Max was projecting or not. Everyone told him he was, but how do we know? How does he know? Only Sam knows. I have seen patients act so convincingly they could win an Oscar! The best liars and gaslighters, those who construct their own reality and then make a winning case for it, leave the listener doubting their own perceptions and beliefs. People lose faith in their own sense of reality. This can drive you crazy.

When Max spoke, every part of me believed him. He was so confident in his assertions, so convincing. When Sam spoke, I knew she was telling the truth, her protestations of innocence were so genuine. Her plea of being falsely accused was so credible. Isn't it great to have two sides of a story?

If Max turns out to be right, then we would have to call him intuitive and seeing beneath the surface, not projecting, not paranoid or delusional. It is not for me, as therapist, to be the ultimate judge of the truth of Max's belief. I'm not a court or a detective and I didn't know whether Sam had cheated or not. I did believe, however, that Max was expressing his intense feeling of betrayal, he was so sure. That is how he felt, regardless of what Sam had or had not done with anyone else, sexually, or otherwise. There was something underlying his sense of betrayal, but it was unclear where that came from—her, or him, his past, her present, or both,—or neither. I can imagine some readers might judge Max as just another dominant male puffing up his alpha chest. I did wonder, myself.

The shift from relating to use involves the destruction of the projective object. In this example, if Max is wrong, what needs to be destroyed is what he put there. Yet, his definiteness allowed no scope for the possibility of him being wrong—how could he be so sure?

In the Winnicott quote above, the reference to "placing the object outside the area of the subject's omnipotent control" can be seen clearly in the example of Max and Sam. He was determined to control her and succeeded to some degree. She grew so oppressed and fearful of his ferocious allegations that she became inhibited and self-conscious. She wouldn't even smile at another person in Max's vicinity as she anticipated a charge of flirting or worse, having had sex with that person.

The object that needs to be destroyed to relinquish omnipotent control is Max's fixed belief that Sam has been cheating behind his back. In this example, trust was shattered, making it impossible for these two to stay together as a couple, whether he was right or not.

> Max and Sam separated after a period of oscillating, together and not-together, on-again/off-again. A year later, we discovered the "truth". Sam confessed to having cheated sexually with both a woman and a man (on separate occasions). Max had appeared delusional and almost psychotic in his fixed beliefs, but these had reflected the measure of hurt, betrayal, and disappointment he felt. His accusation was basically correct, though it had sounded over-the-top. Sam had concealed it from everyone. She offered to confess if he would stop talking to other people about her, stop bad-mouthing her, and stop referencing her on social media, something Max had done constantly much to Sam's distress. He punished her mercilessly until she confessed. Once she did, he did stop, feeling vindicated for being right.
>
> But did she make up that confession to get him off her case?

This example gives a sense of how difficult it can be to analyse what is projective and what is real. There is a power struggle for control both ways. Sam's confession affirmed Max's narrative such that he never questioned it, never doubted it was the "truth". If Sam came to see me privately, I would not be surprised if she said "I just couldn't take it anymore, so I told him what he needed to hear. It worked too, it put an end to his harassment." Sometimes, we never get to know the truth. Did she? Or didn't she? Could it be "double-bookkeeping"?[59] One story for him and another story for me? Only Sam knows.

---

[59] Here, I am using the term more in its original context of accountancy referring to the dodgy practice of keeping two sets of books, one for a desired representation and another for actual transactions. Double bookkeeping in psychiatry usually refers to a person with delusions not concerned by discrepancies or inconsistencies between consensual reality and their own delusional reality. (See, especially, Sass, 1994, pp. 21, 43.)

Destroying an object is what lets it be

Objects have their own, independent existence, their own *being*, if allowed. If you are a mature adult (and I don't mean "old") and you still like to cuddle up to a stuffed animal at night, if that gives you comfort and soothes the anxiety of being on your own, I see no problem with that. When "object" refers to other people, however, it becomes more important for them to be allowed to be separate, as free from projections as possible, or at least to be a willing partner in what they come to mean to you and accepting of your need of them.

The above example raises questions. If Sam hadn't been unfaithful and Max didn't have good reasons to suspect her of infidelities, if he could destroy the object of his mind—that is, his fixed belief in seeing her that way—could they have continued to have a good, healthy, loving relationship? They had been passionate in happier days. Where did his idea come from? He thought he could "see it" when he looked at her with other people. Had his perceptions of her formed a creative apperception that was mistaken to the point of delusion? A case of mistaken identity? Or was he seeing something that was there and being denied, seeing through her?

What needs to be destroyed is what you have turned this person into for your own purposes (apperception), such as *a cheater* (assuming they are not), *a goddess, a hero, a legend, or a villain*, and so on. What needs to survive is that entity or person, as they are, in their own right. That means things and people cease to be what you want them to be, the object of your desire and (mental) construction (even if you turn them into something you really wish they weren't—someone that has betrayed you). Narcissism is relinquished in the process and destroying the object is necessary if a "real" relationship is to become possible. Of course, it helps if your partner speaks truthfully.

Again, mentalization is the psychoanalytic and developmental term for understanding the mental world of others and yourself. It depends upon those others being sufficiently benign and reflective—childhood development depends on this—and similarly for further development in adults (Fonagy, Gergely, Jurist, & Target, 2004, p. 256). But not everyone is benign or reflective.

> Seeing is believing.
> Or does what you believe colour what you see?

Destruction of an object can be met with a challenge. Sometimes what goes on in the mind gets acted out. So, in therapy, a client in the process of destroying his or her therapist (as object) in their mind (destroying their idea of the therapist, an idealised or projected view) attacks the therapist verbally, feels disappointment or resentment, grows critical and becomes aggressive, directly or indirectly. Initially, the patient who asked if I was angry at him got angry at me for being angry at him (as he thought) until he could see his projection. My calmness was a better rebuttal than a reactive defensive denial. It was easier for him to see that I was not angry—a pre-reflective space—than think about whether he believed my claim of not being angry.

Echoing Chapter 4:

> This paradox, once accepted and tolerated, has value for every human individual who is not only alive and living in this world but who is also capable of being infinitely enriched by exploitation of the cultural link with the past and with the future. (Winnicott, 1971, p. xii)

The exploitation of the cultural link with the past and with the future depends upon your *capacity* to destroy the objects of omnipotent control by freeing the objects of your perception from what you want them to be—the object of your desire—to what they are in themselves. (This is phenomenology.) What does this "thing" mean to you? Did you put it there or was it presented from the world? In other words, what you make of something (apperception), including another person in a relationship, is inevitably some mix of who they are, and who they are *to you*.

There is no absolute separation. There is no absolute separateness. There is no self-contained identity of things or people that is fixed and consistent for all and forever. Again, that is the referential sense of meaning. The Buddhist expression for this is *We are not solid*. Is there an objective external reality? Yes, I presume so. Can you ever get to it in its purest form? No, I presume not.

What can be done is this: clear a space in yourself for your perceptions to unfold without prejudice or preconception, without omnipotent control, and without a pre-determined (fixed) idea as to what it, the object, is or what it means. (This is mindfulness in practice.) Notice your biases and remove them or at least suspend them. What your perception has meant to you before (apperception) may or may not be consistent with what it means to you now. Then, the cultural link with the past and future comes into view and can thereby be exploited for your benefit and, potentially, others' enrichment. We will see more of what this means in a moment.

Perhaps to be totally free from preconceptions and omnipotence is something akin to enlightenment. I don't think we can be absolutely free. If anything, this tug-of-war between what you take things to be and what they are—*this most difficult thing*—is the process of transitionality that occurs between you and the world, through your interactions. It is a negotiated process that goes on from birth to death. It starts with your earliest orientation and involves regular reorientation. The more you succeed, the more enriched you become, the more creativity you develop, and the *fuller* your capacity for meaning-making is. In the pursuit of mental health, this is key.

The comprehensive destruction of the object, omnipotently conceived, creates the condition of the possibility of love. You have to destroy your (idea) of your lover in order to love the person of your lover. To be clear—it is not the person that is destroyed but your concept of who that person is. This allows your partner to emerge in their "isness", as they truly are, changing and evolving, as they go, through the coursing of time. We mustn't leave ontology, *the logos of being*, out of mental health.

Maybe Sam cheated because Max imposed his rigid idea of her upon her, thus failing to destroy his internal object-in-himself, such that he could let her be, let her be her, and so love her, for herself and in the process, allow her to love him without his brutal domination. Maybe she had to destroy his idea of her? I can only speculate.

> Love proceeds as projections recede.

Put the other way around:

> The fixed idea is the death of love.

As you develop a capacity to use objects free from your projections of them, you assume a position of greater separateness from them. This is what separateness means. From there, difference is the *sine qua non* of relationship, of exchange and intersubjectivity, even if never absolute. Allow the other to be other. In practice, this means the differences of others, of objects, of the world, are welcomed, even celebrated. How far is this attitude from wanting someone to be the way you want them to be? Or perhaps: to be like you? Or perhaps: to like you?

In couples therapy, often one party wants the other to be something more, better, different, than they are. If your partner could just change a bit, become something more akin to your own architecturally designed blueprint of what you want, then you would be happy in the relationship, and all would be well. Indeed, many people *try* to become what their partner wants. This is not unreasonable and could even be useful, to a degree, for a relationship to work. The risk is that by going too far towards what the other wants and away from yourself, you fall (back?) into the false-self mode.

Requiring a partner to change, fulfil their potential, be a better person, or change their character beyond what they are capable of, is an approach that leads to dissatisfaction and disappointment in yourself and to feelings of inadequacy and rejection in your partner. How long can a person sustain a position of not being themselves? Or trying to be what they are not?

Sometimes, one person believes the other person would be more "themselves" if they were more as the first prescribes. How could this be authenticity?

Taken to its worst extreme, the wish for someone to be different—as opposed to allowing *their* differences—and more so, to pressure them to *be* different, can result in a feeling of annihilation. By annihilation, that person *feels* it has become impossible to be who they are. This is an untenable position, akin to not existing. It also creates an existential vacuum (and you know where that goes). The feeling of annihilation is often accompanied by the loss of hope; energy drains away, leaving depression, deadness, or numbness in its wake. Control from outside may be comprehensive. Compliance and acquiescence are required as a survival strategy. Suicide would be symbolic, as the subject has already been killed. Without choices, Rumi's notion of strength is lost, its possibility systematically dismantled. Taken to its extreme, total acquiescence is an abdication of "selfhood" and, as such, is a formula for a psychotic condition.

Such an untenable position can leave your sense of yourself coalesced with the sense of yourself that a dominant other has, their concept of you. In that con-fusion, there is little option other than to become "a mental patient". Overcoming psychological "annihilation" involves the birth—or re-birth—of the "self" as a separate and authentic person. In the process, the identification of being a mental patient suffering from a pre-defined diagnosis of a psychopathological syndrome needs to be destroyed. That happens through the movement of transition from object relating (the concept of mental illness) to object use (a functioning person free from the stigma of *having a mental condition*). That is where therapy is needed. Such a rebirth occurs through the cultivation of a capacity to use objects through transitional experiencing such that you can function in the world without the risk of being subject to the pathologising judgements of mental health professionals. The object *you have a medical condition and so are mentally unwell* needs to be destroyed in favour of an emerging self-concept such as *you are okay as you are* (especially if you are functional enough to take care of yourself). Otherwise, you can wind up in a locked ward and therapy never begins. And unless therapy can begin, it can never end.

Being medicated out of existence sustains the annihilation that brought you there in the first place.

By contrast, the destruction of the object (how you are defined by others) is conducive for possibilities of meaningful relating and living. There needs to be separateness, especially as you grow up, from your parents and siblings, through your adult relationships; from fusion, through confusion, to de-fusion. The destruction of internal objects opens the way for external objects to come into view. Then objects can be used, not fused. You can live outside the domain of fantasy. You can make things and do things. Creativity is possible, often spontaneous. Meaning emerges. Otherness plays before you in the playground of social intercourse. It could be fun.

Better to be out in the playground of the world than confined inside the enclosure of an institutional ward.

Celebrate destructiveness

Babies' and children's play often involves destructiveness and a blatant pleasure in it. Blocks are piled up, but the real fun is in smashing them down. Games often involve killing. Think about modern gaming; how much of it involves fighting, overpowering, killing, slaughtering, exploding, smashing to bits a virtual opponent. The destructive tendencies of adolescence (now nine to thirty-nine years old) are something that society tends to be intolerant of even though they are essential for emotional growth. Tagging and spray-painting are examples of how young people (usually) can make amazing, artistic creations but also be destructive in where they place them. Public and private property can be defaced or, alternatively, disused areas can be brought to life, drab fencing lit up, and playgrounds made user-friendly. I have often wondered how we, as a society, can promote greater value for our young people. What can young people do to be valued?

I cannot help but wonder if the unfinished developmental business of destroying mental objects gets acted out through violence and other forms of destruction as a consequence of the unfinished business of developing a more creative, and more loving, capacity. That is not the sort of destructiveness to be celebrating.

*　*　*

In therapy, when people are struggling with the transition from object relating to object use, the person of the therapist, the therapist's way of practising, and the therapy setting can be attacked. Attack may take the form of verbal criticism, complaint, or protest at the way something isn't right for the client such that the client cannot make use of the situation in a purposeful way. Sometimes, complaints are well founded but, fair or not, destructiveness can be necessary for such clients. To be developmental, such destructiveness must be *survived* by the therapist, which means not retaliating and avoiding the premature termination of therapy. There is an activity that is attempting to place the therapist outside of the omnipotent control of the client, as a person who exists independently of the client's mental possession or construction, their idea of the therapist. This is a vital function of therapeutic work, but at the same time, it threatens the continuation of therapy. It is part of a transitional process that must run its course. Some novice therapists find it challenging.

Therapists must surrender both the gratification of idealisation and the injustice of de-idealisation as clients give up their previous projections. The subsequent insecurity of not knowing where you stand, how you will be regarded, as a therapist, feels risky but is a developmental function of the transitional process. Transcendence requires the relinquishing of control on both sides—that of the therapist and that of the client.

Similarly, when a child wants something that is denied, parents have been shocked to hear their beloved darling children say "I hate you" or, worse still, "I wish you were dead", or the unforgettable "I wish I had never been born!"—it can be difficult to "survive" such destructive attacks. Survive, in this context, means to bear what feels so hurtful, to take the risk of surrendering to it. At these times, retaliation is neither desirable nor productive. Children usually recover their balance and positive connection to parents. There should be some comfort in the thought that these moments are developmental and serve the positive function of children's separating themselves out from parents, a necessary part of growing up.

In a sense, the hostile child is trying to break free from their parent's mental object or concept of who they are, in the attempt to come into themselves as a separate person.

The formulation *destruction of the object* should not be understood as absolute or as occurring in a physical, final, or total way. Again, there is a to-and-fro quality, a movement, and a flux backward and forward from attachment to non-attachment, from security to freedom, from self to other, and back again. It is a negotiation between the way you want it to be and the way it is. Unlike physical development, emotional development and maturation do not occur solely in a linear direction as physical development does.[60] You work with the world as it shows you that you can't always have what you want, but you can have what's possible and what's there.

Object relating can also involve your relation to your history. As the present unfolds, you may never be completely free of mental activity involved in the conceptualisation of your history or your insights about the past. Nor should you be, necessarily. Many feel a driving need to reconcile their memories of the past, to understand what happened, to interpret what it means. There is a sorting out of what belongs to you, your concept of the past and what you've been told—can you be confident it is accurate? Or is it all just a story? Stories of the past have a way of changing in the future. Such stories are subject to revision with the passage of time.

Therapists need to help patients move through this, to move from their more urgent preoccupations with the past and what it means, to a coming-to-terms with what can be known and what must remain unknowable. There is so much uncertainty that has to be lived with.

Many people feel that their very identity depends on what *really* happened. What if you can't ever know?

It can be helpful to let go of explanations, definitions, and versions of "reality"—all abstract mental constructions that come from somewhere or someone and are subject to distortion. The transition needed is from living in and through a conceptual "reality" populated by "objects",

---

[60] Even ageing does not purely follow the sequencing of years passing that make up the measure of our age. People who are regressed or under-developed often appear (and act and feel) younger than their age. After a bout of severe illness, we can age by a giant leap. A colleague of mine who was sixty always looked and seemed like forty until a severe bout of flu (not Covid-19!). After that, she looked and seemed more like seventy.

in a constructed history: his story, her story, a non-binary story—to living in the practical world in the unfolding present. Whatever happened, you are you, here, now.

> Think of a recurring story, such as a narrative you tell yourself—and ask yourself: *How does this serve you? What affect does it have on you? Is this story the same as one from your past?*

Is your narrative a prison you remain locked in?—a sentence, a prison sentence. Does it discourage you from trying? Does it rationalise your lack of success? Does it perpetuate your subordination? Is it holding you back? Ensuring you remain stuck?

A capacity for creative living grows by destroying the most thought-about mental objects of your attachments in the past and inner narratives in the present. This allows things, people, relationships, activities to mean something to you without their having to remain a certain way, anchored in a fixed position. Your relationships are open, not set in concrete or foreclosed by meanings that remain static and solid. It also means that your attachments can have a somewhat fluid quality because you understand that everything and everyone is in flux—including you. Things change and come to an end.

> You can still find meaning in the world even when you lose what meant the world to you.

Destruction becomes the unconscious backcloth for love of a real object; that is, an object outside the area of the subject's omnipotent control.

Study of this problem involves a statement of the positive value of destructiveness. The destructiveness, plus the object's survival of the destruction, places the object outside the area of objects set up by the subject's projective mental mechanisms. In this way the world of shared reality is created which the subject can use, and which can feed back other-than-me substance into the subject. (Winnicott, 1971, p. 94)

The word "feed" means you can be fed by the world, if you can let it be, as it is. What is there can be nourishing if you can receive it without having to make it into something else. And that is cause for celebration.

Development is also self-discovery through destruction of the object and destruction of the apperceptions that keep you closed. Self-discovery happens through the perceptions that open you up. Closeness rather than closedness.

The "self" in "self-discovery" only makes sense as a concept in relation to "world". There can no more be a self without a world than there can be a baby without someone to care for that baby, the baby's first world outside the womb. World means self and others. Self must involve others, so self-discovery is also other-discovery and world-discovery, at once, just as the discovery of otherness generates self-discovery. It may seem odd that the greatest possibilities for creativity lie in your capacity to destroy your conceptual objects.

> "Destruction" makes fun possible,
> you don't know what will happen.

It is these very objects that litter the landscape of your experience, clog your consciousness, obstruct receptiveness, and prevent you from being fully present to the flow. Clearing away the debris opens the way for the possibility of true mindfulness, or perhaps better still: worldfulness.

Part III

Towards meaning-fullness

CHAPTER 10

Meaning's emergence in potential space

… ambiguity is of the essence of human existence,
and everything we live or think
has always several meanings.
Maurice Merleau-Ponty

Potential space and transitional objects

In *Playing and Reality* (1971) Winnicott puts forward the ambiguous concept of potential space. He is never clear as to what he means by it. He talks around it. Perhaps it has several meanings, as Merleau-Ponty says. As I understand it, potential space is neither internal nor external, it is neither your own psychic space, felt to be inner, nor belonging to the world, felt to be outer. It is a gathering, an occasion for meeting. It is the ground of potential connection. It is an opportunity. Potential space is the condition of the possibility of connection. An example clarifies what sounds complicated:

> When mother leaves the room, a potential space opens up for the baby through the mother's presence and then absence. If baby cannot make use of potential space, baby becomes anxious and cannot continue playing.
>
> Baby can make use of the potential space by continuing to play without undue anxiety, baby can get interested in something in the room. There is no need for baby to get preoccupied by mental activity that revolves around worrying when will mother return. How long can baby continue to use the space of mother's absence? The answer

could be measured in terms of X number of minutes and will vary from one occasion to another.

For the anxious baby, difficulty with this process should not be regarded as a developmental failure but rather depends upon age and stage of development. There is always context. Sometimes, whether baby or adult or in-between, we are more needy than other times. The young baby or even toddler may simply not be "there" yet. As adults, we need to catch up, developmentally, if we are still not there, yet.

In a sense, the baby that can make use of potential space continues to feel connected, to feel a sense of mother's presence despite her absence. There is a separation that is not a separation because this baby can be separate and autonomous for a period of time. Here separateness means connection. This can pertain equally to adults who can remain connected to a partner even though the partner is away.

How is this capacity developed? We know from both parenting that has worked and psychotherapy that has worked that there is an experience of trust and reliability, of safety and of care, and of attention and love, that breeds confidence, internalised as a secure sense of self with a relatively peaceful mind and relaxed body. This is a good basis for a secure attachment, itself the ground for potential space. By contrast, when dependency fails, there is a loss in the child's interest in play, the absorption in the child's activity wanes and there is a corresponding loss of the meaningful symbol. This is a possible crisis.

The idea of potential space affords possibilities for transitional experiencing through play which leads to possibilities for cultural experience. In both the play space of children and the cultural play space of adults, there is a need to separate out what is "me" from what is "not me". If you are only in the "me" position, you find something of yourself in the world, but then there is no potential space for meaning to grow. This is like a fusion of self and world. If the world refers to another person, then the merger is between self and other, or an overlapping of selves, where other is taken to be the same as the self or an extension of self. This is another way of describing narcissism, or at least a narcissistic tendency.

Where separateness occurs, potential space emerges, and connection becomes possible.

> Separateness separates us
> while making connection possible.

For the small child, the transitional object is called the first "not-me possession". In this expression, we can see a movement from object relating to object use, as previously discussed. The advent of the transitional object is the child's first use of a symbol and first experience of play, as far as we can observe and identify it as such. The attitude of the observers, caregivers, or parents of the children also makes an essential difference. Posing no challenge as to where this object originates from and how it comes to have meaning, and be endowed with value, allows its meaning and value to exist and to grow. There can be oscillation between object relating and object use and back—best not to interfere with this process as it unfolds.

According to Winnicott, the transitional object is

> a symbol of the union of the baby and the mother (or part of the mother). This symbol can be located. It is the place in space and time where and when the mother is in transition from being (in the baby's mind) merged in with the infant and alternatively being experienced as an object to be perceived rather than conceived of. The use of an object symbolises the union of two now separate things, baby and mother, *at the point in time and space of the initiation of their state of separateness.* (1971, pp. 96–97, original emphasis)

If baby and mother are psychologically merged, they are not separate and, strictly speaking, not connected. At the point of the initiation of separateness (object use), now a union of the two is possible. This is a different state than a merger or fusion. The union of two people implies a unity.

That said, I find it questionable to say that the symbol can be located at a place in space and time. How? This is a theoretical assertion. We can see the baby's use of a transitional object. And we can infer that this use corresponds to a transition in baby's mind from mother being a concept or object to being a separate, independent entity to be perceived. But here, Winnicott explains baby's experience and presumes to know what it means. I can see no way of determining a precise location in time or space. We can't know, for certain; it is elusive. While I can see no point in space or time that can be identified with confidence as the initiation of baby's separateness from mother, I agree that the use of the object *symbolises* or stands for this movement towards psychological separateness.

The cultural experience of adults

This transition (from merged to separate/connected) also refers to the cultural experience of adults. Cultural experience becomes possible, and more so, desirable and enlivening, once there is movement from mind to world. It begins with play, as indicated earlier, and is located *between* mind or self and world, being neither wholly "in" one nor "in" the other. Cultural experience occurs between you and the environment in the middle ground. Cultural experience partakes of shared traditions, practices, and activities that are meaningful, by which you are "fed" and can contribute.

Of course, it means much more than this. Examples range from sporting events to going out to restaurants, from music concerts to adventures in travelling abroad, from studying towards a degree or learning a trade, to going boating, and so on. These activities exist within a culture and vary from one culture to another. By "fed" I mean a metaphysical sense of nutriment and enjoyment that arises through the shared experience if you can take it "in" and *metabolise* it.

The initiation of separateness (between self and world) is the middle ground or intermediate space, as it is called, but there is no physical *place* where it happens. It is a potential space through transitional experiencing as it provides opportunities for growth in your formation as a person, your separateness, and your capacity for object use, a true sense of relationship, creativity, and cultural experience.

To use potential space depends upon your capacities developed from early experience, especially through transitional experiencing, given the right environment and conditions.

Yet, mothers and caregivers are never perfect, and it is just as well that they are not. It is out of the fallibility, the shortcomings, the "failures", in total care that potential space is born and is used by babies depending upon their own capacities and affinities. And this pertains not *only* to babies. Example are needed:

1) Mum puts a spoonful of food that is too hot in her baby's mouth. It burns, baby screams, looks a little shocked, offended, and cries with tears of pain and insult.

   The potential space emerges if the child has an opportunity to realise that mum did not mean to do this. *It was an accident.* Because mums are fallible and yet can remain "good-enough", every child must grow to understand that an event like this one was a mistake and neither a deliberate injury nor caused by baby's own omnipotence.

2) Dad's car breaks down on the way to collect his child from day care. This child is four years old and not a baby. Dad phones the day care centre and says mum will do the collecting but there will be a delay.

   Here, the child has an opportunity to realise that departures from the usual pattern happen. Even reliable dads can fail to turn up. Children in this situation have an opportunity to self-soothe, to manage their anxiety and to occupy themselves while waiting in this potential space.

3) I forget that I have a regular therapy appointment for a patient at 3 p.m. on Tuesdays and offer that space to someone else. Both people turn up at once, but I can only see one. I feel I should see the one whose regular appointment time it is. The other is disappointed and perhaps wonders if it means something that I double-booked. I can see the other at 4 p.m.—a one-hour wait.

   There is a potential space for the one who waits to realise that therapists are human and make mistakes, and to manage their feelings about it. There is a free hour to do something else, unplanned, a creative opportunity. Will this person use the hour fruitfully and give value to the time, even if only to spend it thinking how best to use their session? Or will they stew in feelings of rejection, disappointment, and resentment? (They'll probably play with their phone!)

   Maybe my forgetting the regular appointment and double-booking does mean something? I'm prepared to look at that.

I felt guilty and annoyed with myself for the oversight. My patient did not capitalise on the opportunity to make me feel guilty (guiltier than I already felt for making her wait for an hour). Rather, she said she was able to make good use of the time because she arrived not really knowing what she wanted to discuss in her session and now she does. This is a perfect example of a potentiated space. She remained positively connected to me, thereby overcoming the annoyance, resentment, or rejection she could well have felt. She could have assumed the moral high ground, asserted a righteous sense of power, and degraded me. She did have a right to complain. What serves her best?

Making experience fresh

Babies find intense experiences in their own personal space. There is a feeling of a first-time-ever quality. Such experiences become charged with energy and meaning and are directed towards various symbols. One of my granddaughters (age three) unravelled a roll of purple plastic rubbish bags and wrapped Granny and myself up in it, tied us up, and delighted in securing our position (forever) just as she was about to leave with her dad, my son. This was a symbolic gesture that I understood as "Stay right there, don't move, I want you right where I can find you, until I come back next time."

The symbol stands for something. You may not know what, which is also okay. The important thing is that the symbolic has been initiated, and it is the initiation into symbolisation that gestates into the birth of meaning. It *means* something to this child, at this time. Meaning is emerging, evolving. When it isn't allowed to emerge, it can become an existential vacuum in time. And that, in turn, can grow to become an emergency.

> When meaning doesn't emerge,
> it risks becoming an emergency.

A common example of disallowing meaning occurs when a parent or carer decides to throw out the dirty, old, ragged, smelly teddy and replace it with a nice, shiny new one. The child is invariably distraught and will not accept the new teddy as a substitute. Children can be very distressed by this turn of events for many reasons. Something that meant everything has been discarded. Their primary carer did not understand how important *this* teddy was to them. What means everything to the child now is shown to mean nothing to their parent. The double loss is irretrievable: of the transitional object (teddy) itself and the sense that what matters to the child matters to the parent. The child is inconsolable, and the parent who has not recognised the object's importance to the child is now impotent to comfort or compensate. The parent may feel regret and guilt, having realised what they've done, while the child appears to be traumatised. *Why wouldn't you be happy with a brand new one?*

For some adults, losing their mobile phone is much the same as the loss of a transitional object to a small child. I thought I had left my phone at the Farmer's Market the other day. I felt total panic—*I run my whole life and work with it!!* I drove back and looked everywhere. When home, I found it on a shelf in my kitchen. Forgot I left it there. Profound relief. I wonder if this is what it is like for a small child and their transitional object?

Returning to the first-time-ever quality: when meaning *does* emerge, it gives experience a freshness and an aliveness, a "feeling of real", that is sometimes all too easily lost in later life. How important this is for mental health. This capacity needs to be sustained so that when you throw open the curtains and see another sunny day, it feels uplifting rather than same-old. And when you make love to your partner for the one-thousandth time, it needs to feel fresh and different for the *eros* of sex to be alive and exciting. For this to be possible, it needs to feel intimate and mean something. It can still have a first-time-ever feeling as you have never been *here* before, at this point in time. This experience is new even though it looks identical to what that fly on the wall has seen before.

Often, we witness what looks like the same play for a child as we have seen before. Indeed, it may look like the exact same experience repeating over and over again. This is far from unusual. Yet this moment is unique in that it feels immediate and intense, like never before, and remains compelling and engaging for the child. This child is present to their experience, into it, entertained, working something out, as happy as the first time, fully absorbed. Adults can learn so much from children.

It is through a creative relation (apperception) to your experience that play comes to life and meaning is available to be found or made. Thus, the familiar feels different even if it is not that different, the repetitive feels new because you have never been exactly in this space and time before. Never.

Freshness involves receptivity, openness, a disposition of wonder, and a willingness to be awed. Experience unfolds in time but never actually repeats in identical ways. It cannot *be* the same even if it *feels* the same. The slightest detail of difference can inspire delight. Engaging with the world regularly on a first-time ever basis engenders care because presence involves a sense of personal and generous investment in what happens. All combined, freshness brings you to compassion and a compassionate relation to the world, all too sorely lacking.

If babies are not given the chance to have such experiences and develop the corresponding capacities to have them,

> then there is no area in which the baby may have play, or may have cultural experience; then it follows that there is no link with the cultural inheritance, and there will be no contribution to the cultural pool.
>
> The "deprived child" is notoriously restless and unable to play, and has an impoverishment of capacity to experience in the cultural field. (Winnicott, 1971, p. 101)

Overcoming the failure to actualise potential space

When dependability breaks down or fails completely, then there is a loss of the precondition for play. The object loses its meaning and so there is a corresponding loss of the meaningful symbol. This may be an underlying basis for the origins of false-self/compliant living, as indicated before, or also of emptiness, depression, and a lack of purpose in living. The possibility of potential space is lost and becomes empty or dead space. It can also become a rather terrifying space, a hopeless space and a helpless one. The feeling of safety is compromised, and anxiety rushes in. The inability to actualise the potential can correlate with the loss of mental health.

Restlessness, fidgetiness, and agitation grows. It becomes impossible to relax. The body registers the split between self and world that reverberates, echoes, and mirrors the split between body and mind. As it becomes charged with the electric intensity of the feeling of threat and lack of safety, your entire physicality, nervous system, musculature tightens up. This arousal is without pleasure. (Reach for your phone?)

What will turn a dead space into a potential space? It is the same for adults as for children. First and foremost, there needs to be an experience of feeling safe and being safe. Then maximum trust and reliability, security and stability, care and love, a suspension of the challenge of direction, definition, explanation, analysis, judgement, or criticism are basic requirements. An empathic attitude helps. Open communication that is not foreclosed by agendas or demands furthers this cause. Respect and trust combine to potentiate a space towards an affective creativity, a creativity with feeling and freshness. Many of the above conditions imply relationship. If there is no one there to support you in this process, then you have to partner with yourself. As adults, we have to be carers of ourselves, though it helps to have someone to support you: a partner, a friend or could be a Developmental Psychotherapist.[61]

Fonagy and his researchers refer to "epistemic trust" which is "defined as openness to the reception of social knowledge that is regarded as personally relevant and of generalisable significance" (Fonagy, Luyten, Allison, & Campbell, 2019, p. 6). In developmental psychotherapy, the therapist registers and reflects back the personal narratives of patients, thus cultivating epistemic trust in the process. In turn, patients are more likely to learn from the therapist and, ideally, develop the capacity to differentiate between those people in their outside lives whose communications are reliable and beneficial and those who are neither benevolent nor trustworthy. This capacity makes a world of difference outside of the consulting room with respect to social relationships that are rewarding or compromising. Relationships—both personal and professional—that allow for epistemic trust open the way for potential space to come into being (Fonagy, Luyten, Allison, & Campbell, 2019).

Attention to potential space is the preparatory work for the emergence of meaning; it is here that people find meaning in themselves, their world, and their lives. This is a basis for

---

[61] One notable source for the idea of developmental psychotherapy came from my experience supervising a group of developmental paediatricians, the specialist branch of general paediatrics.

creative living—potentially—and for mental well-being. Life assumes a different complexion from struggle, anxiety, depression, and lack of motivation. The feeling of confidence in the environment becomes a source of confidence in yourself and vice versa. The feeling of emptiness gives way to a feeling of fullness, meaning-fullness. Possibilities present themselves whereas previously there were none. It is like living on a different planet. Why aren't current mental health practices taking this on board?—it is essential to mental health.

What we find meaningful can still be questionable:

- Is my football team really so deserving of my personal investment or a form of culturally sanctioned madness?
- Is psychotherapy really such a valuable process or do I feel strongly about it because it was valuable for me?
- Is this person, my lover whom I adore, so special or is it just that I see them that way for a time?

I am not posing these questions to be answered intellectually. Intellectualising is not the best approach because you remove yourself from what you are examining, and that fractures your sense of what it means. Research is often fractured by this type of approach, a step removed. What matters is that something *does* matter. It also matters when nothing does.

When the answers to questions like the ones above point back only to me, there is no potential space. All that matters then is self, self-interest, your own agenda (narcissism again). And what has been missed is the value of things in themselves—separate from self—and the potential for fertile exchange.

When the answers to questions like the ones above point back only to the external things, there is still no potential space. "Evidence" supports the view that the football team, psychotherapy, and my lover are all valuable in and of themselves and to others—there is an evidence base—but there is still no potential space. What you bring, your endowment of value, is rendered valueless if you are not a part of the equation. What has been missed is the vital contribution of your involvement, engagement, and relationship, the investment of yourself and the way you contribute to what it means. It needs to be a two-way street.

> Meaning emerges in the "between", in the interplay
> of exchange between self[62] and world.

---

[62] My frequent use of "self" should not be understood as a unified entity that remains the same. The term "self" is highly socially constructed; I employ it as a kind of shorthand, a term that stands for "you". I use it like a pronoun. Similarly, "world" stands for your world, people, activities, environment—not the planet Earth. World is also not

A "between" indicates the existence of two separate "things" though each belongs to the other and, to some degree, each is constituted by the existence of the other. (Think yin and yang.)

The question of where meaning comes from (Winnicott's paradox) protects this potential space of the "between" insofar as the question remains unanalysed and unanswered; it needs to remain ambiguous. "Interplay" means it is not about the object—the football team, psychotherapy, or lover—but how they are used, your relation to such objects. In this context, the word "used" should not be understood in a strictly utilitarian sense but rather as a quality of your relationship to the "things" that matter to you and not the pejorative sense of *I feel used*. In this regard, think about how you *use* your:

- life partner
- children
- parents
- friends
- pets
- hobbies
- home
- work
- colleagues
- money
- free time
- mobile phone(!)
- websites
- body and mind
- God, if you have one
- And anything else that matters to you.

What is your relation to these "things"? What do you contribute? What do you receive? How are *you* used?

Where do you dwell?

Most of us, I assume, dwell in some *place* in ourselves. Place is a metaphor for mental state or state of mind. In psychiatry, the term "mental state" refers to a person's emotions, thoughts, and behaviour. The Mental State Examination follows a set protocol used for assessment by

---

a unified entity, static and constant in form and function. The interplay between self and world is a movable feast, potentially.

psychiatrists. This is not what I'm referring to. I am thinking about your typical mental activity, which is largely patterned and recurring, largely consistent and would probably be familiar to most people. It is not the same every moment but within a range of variation your mental state—the place where you dwell—is probably familiar to you. If I ask: "Where are you right now?" I'm not asking about your city or geographical location. I'm asking where you are in your mind, *in* yourself. In a rather extreme example:

> I was once referred a patient by a psychiatrist who had worked with him in twice-weekly psychotherapy for two and a half years. The psychiatrist felt he had gotten nowhere. This was distressing because his patient, Ted, had made numerous suicide attempts, was self-harming, often psychotic, and had hurt himself badly on occasions, nearly fatally. This was also the worst case of a spider phobia anyone had ever heard of. Ted thought of nothing other than spiders. He would check under his bed first thing for them, he checked his shoes before putting them on, he would stop in the middle of walking down the road and check his clothes, and so on. He could speak of nothing else; it was the thing that worried him most. He couldn't bear the idea of spiders and felt certain they were all around and threatening.
>
> My psychiatric colleague had analysed many possible notions of what spiders could mean. The spider phobia had taken over Ted's mind and was overwhelmingly oppressive. He thought if he could crack the spider phobia, Ted would surely feel better (this is the problem with preconceptions). Were they like a hand grabbing at Ted? Was the language relevant, someone spying on him? Was something bugging him? Was the spider frightening to others? Did he harbour a hidden fear of something out to get him? Spiders are an ancient symbol of power, used for decoration (on your shield) which was thought to make you invincible to arrows. Was Ted seeking to feel more powerful? Did Ted feel stuck in a web of something: lies, deceit, or mendacity? It went on and on. During their sessions, the psychiatrist's mind became as obsessed with spiders as Ted's was (an example of countertransference).
>
> During my first and only consultation with Ted, in which all I heard about was his phobic attitude to spiders, it occurred to me that as every possible avenue of what spiders might mean had already been pursued, I could follow a different track. I asked him: "So, tell me Ted, what do you think about if you don't think about spiders?" Without any hesitation at all, Ted replied "Oh, I think about how my father sexually abused me every day of my childhood and then I want to kill myself."

This is why trauma-informed therapy is so important. Ted could not deal with what had happened in his childhood and needed a way to avoid thinking about it or talking about it. His spider phobia was his survival strategy, it was the only thing that kept him alive. It was fortunate that Ted was not cured of it, indeed, he couldn't allow himself to be cured of it. It was a life-saver in a wild sea of traumatic memories. The spider phobia was the "place" where

Ted needed to dwell. Its function was to take his mind away from his traumatic memories to something he could (try to) deal with, have control over, and protect himself.

It was possible to send Ted back and give his psychiatrist indications for forming a more "holding" relationship with him. Trauma-informed therapy proceeds first with principles of safety and stabilisation, then processing, followed by integration. An analysis of the defence that keeps you alive, or at the very least, away from unbearable suffering, is not safe. For therapy to work, therapists, whatever their professional identification, need to cultivate the right relation to their post-traumatic patients for therapy to work. This entire discussion of transitional experiencing gives indications about what makes therapy work best, and, in the process, to function as a catalyst for adult development.

For Ted, the spiders were a smokescreen. He needed to know that his psychiatrist could hold him in a safe place—a place free from a *penetrating* analysis—before he could begin to address his trauma, how he had been affected by it, how he coped with that. His phobia functioned to protect him from unthinkable anxiety associated with his memories. With the best of intentions, the psychiatrist had become invasive in his attempts to explain the phobia—a different sort of threat as the one posed by Ted's father, but threatening, nonetheless.

The aim of therapy is not to change the mental state of the patient for them but to cultivate the conditions through which desirable changes become possible, according to the patient's needs at the time. It is better to elicit change than solicit change.

When we look at what spiders *mean* for Ted, this story also serves as an example of the problem of referential meaning as described in Chapter 5. Understanding how a patient uses language is not something to be looked up in a dictionary, or a psychotherapy textbook or psychiatric compendium. It is not as if symbols have a set meaning prior to your use of them. Symbols are highly personal, and contextual. They are also culturally determined but only somewhat generalisable. The micro-culture of an individual patient can vary from the macro-culture of the community at large. Ted's way of object-relating through his preoccupation with spiders served the vital function of protection, his intentional meaning. "Spiders" don't have to symbolise anything. Meaning in therapy is more a matter of understanding than translation.

Meaning is personal. The way every person uses language is personal to them, and then interpersonal in the context of their relationship to others. A person may use words differently, and their terms of reference have different meanings, depending upon who is spoken (or written) to, and the context. To me, Ted was utterly clear that spiders, and his use of them as an object of mind, was the "place" where he needed to dwell. That meant he didn't have to dwell on his traumatic experiences of abuse that involved unbearable pain and, no doubt, confusion about how his father could have treated him that way; how his father could have used him so selfishly and harmfully.

I have a problem with the many this-means-that approaches found in some self-help books. They often pertain to dream analysis or psychosomatic symptoms. If you dream of a tower, it stands for a penis. If you see an elephant in the clouds, it means there is something you cannot forget or can't speak about (the elephant in the room). If you have a headache, it means there is something you don't want to think about. NO, IT DOESN'T! (Sorry for shouting.) It could, but it doesn't have to. Even if these attributions fit, there is something lost from the process of a person coming to what something means for themselves.

I could say to Ted: "Spiders are creepy crawlies that are out to get you" and add "And your father was a creep that was also out to get you, and he did." This becomes cleverness that could be meaningful to him, but is bound to mean less than if Ted were to arrive at his own sense of what spiders mean to him, or to let his preoccupation with them go when he is ready, when he no longer needs to think about them all the time. This probably depends on his ability to process what was done to him and how it affected him, no doubt a very big mountain to climb. This can take many years but sometimes we do see one of the best benefits of therapy, that is when an object (like spiders) or a subject that has preoccupied a patient for hundreds of sessions (like invasive thoughts) no longer needs to be brought up. This is not an omission but rather an issue that has lost its charge. I call this a negative benefit; the benefit is in its absence as an issue or obstacle that was previously a source of stress or distress and dominated a patient's psyche, and the therapy discourse.

One patient had spoken about her mother every session for the past 300 sessions. Here, "mother" should be understood as a most painful and disappointing subject. For the past two sessions, however, she has not mentioned her, except once, in passing—"You know how mum likes to bring over food …" No pain there. I haven't said anything. Imagine if I said: "On a scale of one to ten how much is your mother still an issue for you?" … Huh?

While the story of Ted gives an idea of what I mean by mental state, thankfully most of us don't have to dwell in such a persecutory phobic state of mind. Many people do find it impossible to be with themselves because their mental state is too uncongenial (or worse) and feel imprisoned within that. There are many ways to avoid, postpone, defer, distract, or disengage. Dissociate.

- Can you sit still in silence for an hour? With another person?
- Can you spend time on your own without having to be constantly distracted by social media, some device or screen, headphones to play music, podcasts, chats, texts, streaming news, or some other preoccupation? (There is nothing wrong with any of these things, but can you do without them?)
- Can you meditate?
- Can you relax?
- Can you rest?
- Can you spend an hour paying attention to your breath? Your body? The panorama of sounds in your environment? Or the movement of the clouds while you lie on your back? (There are elephants up there …)
- Can you read or listen to a book or audiobook and stay focused? (Hello, right now!)
- Can you concentrate while you write? A letter? A long email? Such that it makes sense and hangs together?
- Can you hold your thoughts together and in sequence as you speak them?

- Can you lie naked in the dark in a sensory deprivation flotation pod for an hour? And enjoy it? And reach to a deep state of peace?
- Can you sleep? (A proper deep REM sleep!)

Some people have no problem with any of these questions, but many do. Many cannot do any of them at all. Sleep disorders are legion. Many go to great lengths to avoid being with themselves in their own mental state. Some examples are:

- Having a drink (or five) immediately after work
- Smoking a bong or spliff or joint or billy of weed, pot, bud, mull, ganja, cannabis, or marijuana, (or whatever you call it)
- Going straight to the computer, tablet, or device, scanning social media, news, sport, share prices, crypto, fashion, celebrities, whatever
- Texting friends incessantly
- Having your face in your phone walking down the road (oblivious to the cars coming)
- Getting trashed on the weekends (whatever that means: the pub, drugs, trips, getting baked, cooked, drunk, or some combination)
- Porn viewing and compulsive masturbating
- Obsessive house cleaning
- Extreme exercising or gym training
- Binge eating, or the opposite—starving
- Over-relying on medications to alter mood or reduce anxiety
- Over-sleeping
- Financial wheeling and dealing, gambling, over-trading
- Compulsive shopping
- Endless gaming.

I am not judging any of the above and I am no stranger to some of them. Activities like going to the gym and cleaning your house can be perfectly healthy and desirable. I am raising a question about the way you go about it—the use of an object. Is it avoidance? Is there some urgency or need to avoid your mental state or emotional life, or change it?

Many come to therapy looking to find a way out of their mental state. "I don't want to feel like this! Can you fix it?"

1) "Why do I feel anxious when there is absolutely nothing going on that should worry me?"[63]
2) "Today, I woke depressed and haven't been able to shake it."
3) "I've been depressed for months though nothing happened to precipitate it."
4) "I feel so irritable and grumpy for no reason I can think of?"

---

[63] Obviously written before the pandemic!

5) "I just fidget and can't sit still for a moment, my nerves are jangly, like an electric current is running through them, I can't stop my leg vibrating up and down."

6) "I woke crying in the middle of the night. I don't even know what I was dreaming about. And this can happen in the day, too. I can burst into tears without warning. It happened at work last week when I was in a meeting. It is sooo embarrassing."

7) "I had sex with my girlfriend and then as soon as we finished, I felt urgent to go again. So, we did. Even after that I wasn't satisfied. I feel aroused all the time, I just want to keep having sex again and again. Sometimes, I have to do for myself even though we've just done it together, just to try to get some relief."

8) "I am constantly afraid that someone is trying to break in. I know I live in the safest neighbourhood in town, that's why I moved here, but every little noise makes me jump. I imagine there is someone outside the window. I'm in a state of heightened tension that someone is on the roof or is about to burst through the door."

9) "I feel like I am mourning a death, but I cannot place it. There have been no major losses, but I seem to be in a constant state of grief."

10) "I know I had a traumatic childhood but now in my fifties I am still so vigilant. It is as if I am on guard duty 24/7—as if some threat was just around the corner. I scan every room I enter. It is as if I had a radar dish circling over me, always registering any movement or possible threat."

And a different post-traumatic presentation:

11) "I am just so spaced out all the time. I cannot get my mind to focus, even on perfectly simple cognitive tasks I know I am capable of. I can't remember my mother's phone number even though I phone regularly. Yesterday, I forgot my son's best friend's name. I keep forgetting where I put things and I walk into a room and can't remember why. It's as if my whole system has slowed to a crawl."

The best way out of your mental state is by paying attention to it. Usually, there are personal reasons why you feel like that, even if you cannot see them. The reasons can be terribly elusive, though sometimes, once they are visible, they are obvious. When the personal reasons are too elusive or complex, professionals resort to biological explanations: "You have a biochemical imbalance in the brain. It's your hormones, darling."

> ## The best way out of your mental state is into it.[64]

---

[64] This sounds like a contradiction to the previous "break out" that said "Get out of your mind and into the world." The point here of going *into* your mental state is so as not to be stuck there, to work towards being able to get out of it.

For every example above, there were reasons:

1) The anxious patient above had been telling me for weeks that she was increasingly feeling that her partner—the one she had always felt was for life—probably wasn't right for her and not the best choice of someone to have children with. He doesn't like children and doesn't want them, whereas she could not live without a possibility of having them. This will have to be dealt with, but she doesn't know how and cannot face a confrontation.

Anxiety often functions like a wave of noise or the "static" when a radio station isn't tuned in. It covers over your mental functioning like a blanket, making it hard to think or feel your feelings clearly and connect them with their object (the reason). Most anxiety is anticipatory. Underlying reasons are de-coupled from the present but found in an imagined and fearful future. This makes it difficult to know why you feel anxious. It takes over your conscious experience with a nervous charge, as if your finger was plugged into the electric socket. It might be called free-floating, as if it came from the air, but usually there are underlying reasons infused with fear about the future.

2) The example of the depressed person here was me. I'm not often depressed but, on that day, I was. I couldn't shake it or understand why. Things were going well enough. I wanted to know why I felt like that; depression is a horrible feeling. I was reflecting, looking for associations, scanning my inner world for clues but without success. I was having a walk by the sea at sunset time near to where I live. Then I realised the date—it was 12 November 2008. Instantly, I worked out it was the fortieth anniversary of my mother's death. As soon as I made the connection, I started to feel better, depression started to lift. It made perfect sense that I would have a feeling of loss, even though it was such a long time ago. I couldn't get to the feeling of loss because depression was in the way, like a roadblock. Its underlying reason was in the distant past. When I understood why and could connect the feeling of loss with its object, the feeling could be gone through, meaningfully, and hence, lessen towards relief. Our whole psycho-physiological system registers anniversaries often out of our awareness. This is also an example of the importance of symbolisation, making the connection between feeling and meaning, formulating it in words, and then "coming to terms" with it.

The loss was not just of my mother's death. She died at a low point in our relationship. I was sixteen years old, rebellious, defiant, and wild—out of control, really. Unlike my relationship with my father, which improved from that time, my relationship with my mother never had that chance. And that was a significant aspect of the sense of loss.

Sometimes, depression is the consequence of being disconnected from the object of loss, even if the loss happened long ago and you haven't felt depressed about it before.

3) The other depressed person, named Marissa, had been depressed for months and struggled to understand why. When we investigated it in therapy, we discovered that around the time it began, her lover, a woman named Radhika, had revealed that her former partner had contacted her and wanted to get back together with her. This former partner, Claire, was both strikingly beautiful and had a high public profile. Radhika had been disturbed and somewhat unhinged by various psychological games Claire played. Claire had been more than liberal with the truth and often indulged in gaslighting to the point that Radhika began to doubt her own perceptions. Her very sense of reality had been called into question. Radhika fled this relationship and didn't want to go back. In discussing this with Marissa she revealed for the first time just how powerful her bond with Claire had been. She called it "the most powerful relationship of my life".

That meant it was more powerful than Radhika's current relationship with Marissa. Words are so important. I don't think Radhika had intended to make this point to Marissa, who felt shocked and hurt by it.

What surprised Marissa more, however, was how overwhelmed with hatred she felt for Claire and how threatened she felt at the same time. She was not a hateful person and found this emotion intensely disagreeable; "toxic" was the word she used. She felt poisoned, polluted by hate for her partner's ex-partner. Her depression was a suppression, in this case, that avoided the feeling of hatred in herself that she couldn't bear. Once this connection was *symbolised* and, equally, once Marissa could allow her feelings of hatred to be felt, her depression shifted, lessened, became intermittent, and then, with time, waned. She had to come to terms with how she *really* felt—it was more effective than medication, a different form of suppression.

4) The irritable, grumpy person is affected by the hormonal changes the week before her menstrual period. She can never remember it is that time of the month. This happens often, though not every month. Probably, this is primarily a biological issue. However, if she could notice the underlying reason for her irritability, as it is patterned, she would be able to live with it more easily (and so would everyone else), if only she could symbolise it as she felt it coming on.

Women have told me that when they are able to say "I'm feeling pre-menstrual (and this is a bad one)", they fare better in avoiding damage to relationships (including with children). Much of the time, it appears the pre-menstrual woman is already genuinely irritated about something at a personal level and the PMS intensifies and exacerbates the feelings. Symbolising this part of it enables the issues to be addressed (potentially) without a damaging emotional storm.

5) The fidgety person who cannot sit still was about to assume a new role in his company in which he would hold substantially increased responsibility. He had taken a big increase in salary but had doubts as to whether he was up to the task. (Imposter Syndrome.)

6) The person who had been crying for no reason was a passionate crusader to protect the environment to save orangutans in their ever-compromised habitat and dwindling

numbers. She started crying two and half weeks ago. It's important to pay attention to timing. "Wasn't that the time when massive fires were deliberately lit in the Indonesian rainforest by companies and farmers wanting to clear land to plant trees for palm oil?" As soon as I said it, my patient looked shocked—she had found this devastating, a massive setback for her cause—but she was having to put it out of her mind in order to function in the day. She knew instantly this is what had been affecting her and bringing her to tears. Knowing what something means and being able to speak about it initiates movement. That is what the word emotion means: e-motion = outward movement.

7) The man who couldn't be satisfied sexually and was constantly aroused had been raised primarily by a nanny. She had sexually interfered with him in different ways. Throughout much of his early childhood she teased him, stimulated him, and aroused him genitally and anally. She undressed in front of him and organised ways that he could see her bathe, go to the toilet, and stand in front of the mirror in varying degrees of undress. She seemed to take pleasure in this form of sexual play, and he was like a plaything for her. (Obviously not the sense of play espoused here.) As an adult, he had episodes of being aroused and unable to be fully relieved of it, despite much sexual activity. It was *as if* the memory of his nanny and her abuse was never far from his mind (or body). This is post-traumatic. As a child, he was rarely far from sexual arousal and so, as an adult, this carried over even without overt stimulation, or even following a lot of it. His body was perpetually aroused.

8) The paranoid-sounding woman who was constantly preoccupied with the thought that someone was trying to break in had been telling me how lonely she was. Some of her friends had moved away and others seemed less inclined to spend time with her. She had been on dates, but no one was right for her. She longed for company. Her fear of an intruder seemed more like a wish that someone would want to see her so badly, would want to get "into her" (into her heart, in a way) that they would "break in" to her home. Of course, she didn't want someone to literally break into her home. In working together, she came to see her fear as a transformation of a disavowed wish. Once the feeling was acknowledged and made intelligible (symbolised), her fears reduced and were replaced by sadness. This sadness was motivating for her to make some friends, whereas the paranoiac fear had led her to greater withdrawal from people. Her isolation had become like a fortress from which she longed to be rescued.

9) The person suffering grief and loss for no (apparent) reason realised that his long-term dream of being able to overcome his disability was never going to happen. He was paraplegic (paralysed from the waist down) following a childhood accident. He had worked very hard with new technology that held a possible promise of regaining control and movement of his legs. But alas, it wasn't working and didn't look like it was going to. Though he had lived with this for a very long time, he had been holding out hope for a change. The loss of that hope was like a death to him. Here, symbolisation relieved him of false hope but now, new sources of meaningful living would be necessary once he could fully "come to terms" with his disappointment and the reality of his situation.

10) Lastly, trauma often brings in its wake a state of hyperarousal or hypo-arousal. As a child, this man had a mother who could be loving one minute, then without warning, viciously attack him. Once, she bit a hole in his cheek. He never knew in what mood he would find her. His hyperarousal and hypervigilance carried over to his adult life. Ted, with the spider phobia, is also an example of extreme hypervigilance.

11) The woman in the final example—spaced out and forgetful—had been gang-raped as a fifteen-year-old. She wasn't sure this past trauma accounted for her mental state, but I felt she had not dealt with her trauma sufficiently. Such extreme experiences tend to require a great deal of therapeutic work over years. Prospects for recovery are good if the work is undertaken.

The trauma literature is substantial and has come a long way in the past twenty years or so. Suffice to say that clinicians are learning more about what "safety and stabilisation" means for trauma survivors, what "processing" entails, and what is involved in "integration" (see Kezelman & Stavropoulos, 2012, 2019).

It is not hard to see why people in general—all kinds of people—want to change their mental state. Going into the reasons in depth and detail—the current circumstances, the history, and the ways you have been affected—helps to work through such patterns of thinking, feeling, acting, and, especially, suffering. If you want to change your thinking, don't treat it like a machine that requires tools to manipulate it. Your thinking isn't a problem to be solved, a puzzle to be completed, or a maze that requires strategies to find a way out. Your mind is not a machine that needs the right instruments to repair it. It's more therapeutic to recognise that your thinking expresses something about yourself. If you want to change it, go right into it. Running away changes nothing because your thinking follows you. Dwelling where you are is the most effective position from which to move on. Once you are ready, realise what needs to be realised and go through what you must. You have to do the work for yourself—but you don't have to do it *by yourself*.

> Regarding your mental state,
> renovate first,
> then you can move house.

Meaning's emergence

How can you shift your mental state, your psychology, or your personal manner of mental processing, *the place where you dwell*? The idea of potential space is to initiate movement through an experience of greater connectedness. To make use of potential space, you first have to realise there is a potential space—or it needs to be created. Initiating movement out of your mental isolation and towards the world, that is, towards another person, opens the possibility of the "between" of a relationship. It could be a personal or professional relationship, or both, but with different people. Meaningful symbols are created in and through the "between" space of connected relationships.

By contrast, when there is a loss of the meaningful symbol, or an inability to find or create one anywhere, then there is emptiness that corresponds with inaction or inertia, as discussed earlier. You can be (apparently) mentally and physically healthy, that is, free from any diagnosable disorder, and still have no idea what your life is about, or what you are about.

In another language, the locus of your thinking needs to shift from schizoid experiencing where:

- You are looking at the world from behind your eyes.
- You see the world as if on a screen.
- You slip into fantasising, and prefer it to reality.
- You don't really feel in it or a part of it.
- You are full of dreams of who you are, where you should be, and what will happen when you are truly recognised or discovered (the opposite of Imposter Syndrome!).
- You indulge in action dramas in your mind in which you are invariably the hero, fighting off villains and rescuing someone.
- Your experience is often abstracted and divorced from the practical realm.
- You are withdrawn, avoid people, find other people strange, prefer your own solitary company (you might still long for a soulmate).
- You are emotionally underdeveloped and frequently experience childlike reactions to things.
- You feel a fraud, imposter, or like a child, and feel fearful others will notice.
- Life is about getting by, surviving, avoiding conflict, and not being discovered as far as possible.

Schizoid experience tends to be isolated and withdrawn, the locus is interior, such that the possibilities for potential space are lost. There are also many positive qualities in the more schizoid personality type—often there is acute intelligence combined with sensitivity—and anyone can feel like one or more of the above points without necessarily being a schizoid character. *I'm not setting out to diagnose you!*

Whether you are a schizoid character or merely have some schizoid tendencies, the aim is to move the locus of your attention from the fantasy realm of your "inner world" to the physical and social world of meaningful activities and relationships with other people. This movement is the actualisation of potential in potential space, where transitional experiencing and symbolisation come together and give birth to the emergence of meaning.

CHAPTER 11

Beyond Winnicott: "I play, therefore I am"

We are never more fully alive,
more completely ourselves,
or more deeply engrossed in anything
than when we are playing.
Charles E. Schaefer

So far, we have treated *play* as a subjective experience, especially in the context of early child-hood development. To speak of play as a subjective experience refers to an attitude and an activity for oneself—*what play is to me*. For Winnicott, this experience is the basis of creativity, and creativity is an essential part of the capacity to make meaning and grow as a person.

While the subjective experience of play cannot be denied, there is a larger dimension to which Winnicott himself gestures:

> *it is play that is the universal*, and that belongs to health: playing facilitates growth and therefore health; playing leads into group relationships; playing can be a form of com-munication in psychotherapy; and lastly, psychoanalysis has been developed as a highly specialized form of playing in the service of communication with oneself and others. (1971, p. 41, original emphasis)

And ... "playing is itself a therapy" (1971, p. 50). These are powerful statements of human experience, and in making them, Winnicott is not alone. Since antiquity, heavy-weight thinkers have given play a privileged role in human experience. Amongst the pre-Socratics, for Heraclitus, "Man is most nearly himself when he achieves the seriousness of a child at play". For Plato, "Life must be lived as play, playing certain games … singing and dancing" (Huizinga, 2006, p. 97). More recently, the significance of play has been addressed by Hegel, Marx, Nietzsche, Heidegger, Gadamer, and other philosophers.

One of the most striking contributions to the subject is Johan Huizinga's *Homo Ludens: A Study of the Play Element in Culture* (1970, first published in 1938). Huizinga argues that play has been a seminal influence in the formation and development of human civilisation. All play means something beyond its biological function; it is not adequately understood as a psychological reflex, not explained by instinct (Freud) or will (Adler), nor as something that precedes culture. "In play there is something 'at play' which transcends the immediate needs of life and imparts meaning to the action. All play means something" (1970, p. 19). An important source for Huizinga is a passage in the fifteenth letter of Schiller's *Letter on Aesthetic Education* (1795):

> Play allows humans to fulfill their very natures: "man only plays when he is in the fullest sense of the word a human being, and *he is only fully a human being when he plays*" (NA XX, 359/E 131). (Moland, 2021, original emphasis)

Homo Ludens, Man the Player, instead of *Homo Sapiens*, Man who is Discerning, Wise, Sensible (in short, Man the Thinker). In the spirit of this provocative switch, we play upon the famous dictum of Descartes: "I think, therefore I am."

For Descartes, there is an "I" for whom *thinking* is *being*. Following Huizinga, let us say instead: "I play, therefore I am." Here, there is an "I" for whom *playing* is *being*. Simply, being human involves a distinctively human way of playing.[65]

How can play be a mode of *being*? One approach to this question is found in Hans-Georg Gadamer's landmark philosophical work *Truth and Method* (1975, pp. 91–119).[66] For Gadamer, the subjective sense of play has dominated Western aesthetics and philosophy. He examines play and sets out to free the concept from its purely subjective meaning.

In this chapter, I call upon Gadamer to enlarge our understanding of play. My aim is to show how play builds a capacity for creative living and meaning-fullness, and, ultimately, to explore the value of play for therapy itself.

---

[65] Recall the Frankl quote in the epigraph to the whole book: "Step by step I progressed, until I again became a human being." This could be understood as once again able to play freely.

[66] The chapter titled "Play as the Clue to Ontological Explanation" informs my treatment of this subject. I am elaborating my understanding of Gadamer, who was first a student, then a close associate, of one of the greatest philosophers of the last century, Martin Heidegger. Heidegger's thought was a profound influence on Gadamer who is best known for his major work on hermeneutics: *Truth and Method* (1975).

The spirit of play

How seriously should we take play? It is easy to think of play as the least serious thing. We say of something that it is *merely child's play*—too easy for *adults*. Play is what we do when we're not serious!

On the contrary, the fun (enjoyment, pleasure, thrill) we experience in play *depends* on a certain kind of seriousness. The young child is engrossed in play while babbling happily. In the case of adults, for whom play often takes more organised forms (a sporting event, theatre, concert, religious ceremony), there is still an imperative for seriousness. For this to happen, play needs to be taken seriously by the player. Imagine how boring it would be if the players in a sporting event, theatre, concert, or temple, did not take it seriously. If the players just mucked around, hadn't practiced and rehearsed together, *play* would lack intensity, immediacy, and affect. The audience would register a lack of care and investment.

I'm reminded of a Rolling Stones documentary. I was impressed to discover how much work went into the group's albums and performances despite their reputation for drug-taking, partying, and having a wild time (back in the day). When producing a recording, they were perfectionistic and went over and over it until it was right. They wanted their music to outlast their own lives and they took it more seriously than many, which has a great deal to do with their enduring success.

There are occasions, however, when play attracts excessive seriousness, especially when the stakes are high. Naturally, high stakes may be experienced in any form of play (e.g. frisbee-throwing can become competitive disk golf), depending on the disposition of the player, but let me take some examples that resonate in the public domain—namely, international competitive sports such as professional tennis. We witnessed the furore around Serena William's outburst in the 2018 American Open. Earlier: "You can't be serious", screamed John McEnroe to the umpire—but McEnroe was dead serious. Sometimes, having missed a shot, he would fling himself on the ground in a foetal position. After losing a match in a Grand Slam tournament, Goran Ivanisovitch was asked by an interviewer how he felt. Instead of dishing up the usual platitudes—"It was a close game", "I had my opportunities", "My opponent played well"—Ivanisovitch muttered: "I want to kill myself."

Life or death. Sometimes, in such cases, the player is treated as a bad sport or sore loser. I want to approach the matter from a different angle, which concerns the relation of the player to the spirit of play. To explain what I mean by "the spirit of play", consider a personal experience.

> I played basketball during my university days. It wasn't *the real deal of American college basketball*; it was only a little New England league of local colleges. It was serious for me. Our best player, a centre, was formidable and was our team's greatest asset. He was a big bloke, tall, and strongly built, dominating, and intimidating to the other teams. However, he smoked marijuana before each of our most important matches.

I remember vividly the feeling of my heart sinking to the pit of my stomach when our centre turned up visibly stoned. He was happy, but his game became casual and ineffective. We always lost.

He was fine for the less important matches. We had a good team and progressed. We lost *all* the big matches, the ones that mattered most. We needed our centre to perform but he couldn't cope with the pressure. Getting stoned meant he couldn't care less.

I always ended up feeling angry and disappointed (subjective experience). I don't really know why he did that. I suspect he cared too much, felt a burden of expectation, and got anxious before the big matches. Perhaps, for him, it was *too* serious. Being *out* of his head meant he could only get *into* the spirit of play in a limited way (which limited the rest of us!).

In this example, getting into the spirit of play has nothing to do with someone's being a good sport or a bad sport. It concerns something that Gadamer considers fundamental to play itself:

> We have seen that play does not have its being in the consciousness of the attitude of the player, but on the contrary, draws the latter into its area and fills him with its spirit. The player experiences the game as a reality that surpasses him. (1975, p. 98)

It is not only a question of attitude, of subjectivity, or of getting into the correct mindset. It is not really about the "head-space" of the players. It is more a matter of allowing yourself to be drawn into the nature of play itself. Gadamer says we are filled with *its* spirit, the spirit of play and of the game that is being played. This is what our "centre" could not allow in the big matches.

> Play fulfils its purpose only if the player loses himself in play. It is not that relation to seriousness which directs us away from play, but only seriousness in playing makes the play wholly play. (1975, p. 92)

Once again, there is a movement *out* of yourself and into the activity that you are *in*. It moves you. You are "into it". It infuses you with its spirit, its energy, its dynamic involvement. And by so doing, you experience the game as a reality that surpasses yourself. This surpassing has a transcendent quality (remember Frankl: self-transcendence). It is a lifting of yourself first to yourself and then beyond yourself by being infused with spirit. Spirit is life, breath, movement, flow, being—and as such, spirit is meaning. There is something "happening" here that is unfolding, a happening of self in a world full of meaningful possibilities.

> Meaning comes into being through
> the spirit of play and the play of spirit.

The theme of *movement* recurs throughout this book. The ideas of development, creativity, play, meaning, and therapy are all expressions of a movement from one position to another (such as from merged to separate, object relating to use). Understanding this is essential, but there is no substitute for action.

The player knows that they are playing and that it is *only* a game. You are not lost in play if you are self-conscious or thinking *it's only a game*. My basketball friend could not get lost in the play when it mattered; he had to get "out-of-it" instead of into it. If anything, one purpose of play is to get out of your self, in a funny way of speaking, out of your mind. Out of your mind and into the game. Or out of your mind and into living. There is a movement. Too much thought removes us from the spirit of play. When he smoked, my friend got too far into his mind—in a spaced-out way—to be able to play properly. Lost in his head, he could not take his place on the field of play. He couldn't move properly.

> ## When play works, it takes you out of yourself.

Instead of losing your head, you must lose yourself in play. This is central to Gadamer's aim to make the subjective experience of play for the player subordinate to play as the thing itself. The structure of play absorbs the player into itself.

Gadamer says: "The being of all play is always realisation, sheer fulfilment, energeia[67] which has its telos[68] within itself" (1975, p. 101). In Greek, *energeia* means work, even though it looks like the word "energy". This reference suggests work can be play and play can be work (as we said in Chapter 7). Or: there is play in work and work in play. Telos usually refers to a built-in goal or purpose. So, the aim or goal of the being of play is in the doing of it, itself, for its own sake. Play, like the work of art, is autotelic praxis, praxis-for-its-own-sake. It realises itself in being (presencing). Playing is made real through playing—it sounds circular—and so too is the player absorbed in it. There is no end, only the "make-believe goals" that are imposed by us:

> The self-representation of human play depends, as we have seen, on the behaviour which is tied to the make-believe goals of the game, but the "meaning" of the latter does not in fact depend on achieving these goals. Rather, in spending oneself on the task of the game, one is, in fact, playing oneself out. The self-representation of the game involves the player's achieving, as it were, his own self-representation by playing, i.e. representing something. Only because play is always representation is human play able to find the task of the game in representation itself. (1975, p. 97)

---

[67] *Energeia* (ἐνέργεια) is an important Greek technical term in the works of Aristotle. His coinage indicates something being "in work". It is the etymological source of the modern word "energy".
[68] Telos is Greek for purpose, end, or goal.

A tough quote. I met Gadamer, and Laing, as a student. I was not up to criticising their thought then, but I would like to have a word with them now, if only I could.[69] I would ask Gadamer what he means by "in spending oneself on the task of the game, one is, in fact, playing oneself out". There seems to be a play on words here. To spend oneself is to be spent—exhausted. The same is true of "playing oneself out". At the same time, to play yourself out is to play out of yourself. Paradoxically, to come *out* of yourself is to come *in* to yourself. This is true to experience. You come out of yourself through your absorption and thereby come into yourself through your immersion in an activity. A simple example:

> I'm not much of a pianist but there was a time when I devoted myself to learning and playing the piano. I practised for around six hours each day. My music instructor at university gave me the key to the auditorium so I could use the Steinway Concert Grand Piano—thankfully, there was no audience. I played myself out and felt joyful through being wholly immersed in making music. I never felt more myself than when I was playing even though I knew I would never be Concert Grand material.

It became a game to play and play and play. The goals of the game were "make-believe" and the playing of it sheer fantasy (schizoid?).[70] I walk out on to the stage of Carnegie Hall to rapturous applause. Then I bring the house down with my perfect rendition of the Chopin Ballade in G Minor (though it was always far from perfect in reality).

Is this what Gadamer means by "representation"? I was playing the game of concert pianist. Every form of play positions the player in a role such as hero, saviour, villain, ruler, destroyer, competitor, rock star, champion, or arts legend, and so on. Is this not illusion? Play represents the task of the game while the "make-believe" goals allow us to entertain a certain sense of meaning. The highest score wins or the first with no cards left in their hand wins, or whatever. Wins what? Often nothing other than wearing the mantle of winning for a few brief moments. Then we play again.

---

[69] In 1980, I attended the *Collegium Phaenomenologicum* in Perugia, Italy, for a summer devoted to the study of Heidegger. Gadamer attended one session. One of the academics got into an argument with him over a point of interpretation of what Heidegger really meant by a passage in his great work *Being and Time*. The argument raged back and forth until Gadamer (finally) played his trump card. "I know I'm right because Heidegger told me so!", making any further argument pointless. Or was he just playing?

[70] What is the difference between my practicing six hours per day and an obsessional disorder? Maybe there was a touch of obsessionality but for me it was a meaningful activity. There was a choice. I did it because I wanted to and enjoyed it. *It was compelling but not compulsive.* In obsessional disorders, there is a have-to quality. The activity is mechanical, repetitive, and obligatory. It is as if the activity demands to be done—*go inside and check the stove!*—whereas for me, there was no demand in it at all. It was pure pleasure, an expression of my desire. I couldn't wait to get into the auditorium and play. We get into all kinds of difficulties and confusions when someone calls a meaningful and desired activity, even if oft repeated, an obsessional symptom. Such is the problem of *pathologising*.

However, the significance of play does not depend upon achieving the "make-believe" goals of the game. Being so absorbed in play makes it meaningful. You become yourself (self-representation) through the act of playing, especially if play is more free-form and creative. There is a coming into being, an aliveness, a birth of self that occurs through play. It is not just being born into yourself but more than that, a being born of your self into the world. I play, therefore I am.

I will never be a concert pianist. But I can play.

Living as play

In *Man's Search for Meaning* (2014), Viktor Frankl makes a challenging statement: "Life is a game that plays us." If this is so, we are at a considerable disadvantage because we do not know the rules of the game. On the face of it, we are merely playthings of an arbitrary power. If we are dealt a bad hand, what can we do except throw up our arms in weary resignation and lament the capriciousness of fate?

By no means. For Frankl—a concentration camp survivor—meaning can be found in even the most acute suffering, and finding it depends on establishing a proper relationship with life. An example comes to mind:

> The father of a friend of mine was an elderly man in his late eighties and as fit as a fiddle. He was an avid reader (he was trained as a Classical scholar) and had a passion for gardening. One day when working in the garden he slipped and fell on a low picket fence. A picket pierced his eye—a dreadful injury. He lost that eye and for a long time was unable to read.
>
> My friend was abroad when he heard the news and anxiously rang his father to commiserate and ask how he was managing.
>
> His father replied: "One day a rooster, the next day a feather duster."

This was a witty response and for that reason, I believe, a healthy one. Mental health depends more on coming to terms, adjusting to what happens, than succumbing in misery. Rather than capitulate to life's game, he embraced it. While he may not have found meaning in the horrible event, he played with it creatively through wit. Charlie Chaplin: "To truly laugh, you must take your pain, and play with it!" Yes—if you can! On the other hand, before him, the eighteenth-century philosopher and writer Voltaire said: "God is a comedian playing to an audience too afraid to laugh." In his case, my friend's father wasn't afraid to laugh. He entertained a properly playful relation, both to life and to himself, even his permanent injury.

With the above in mind, I want to consider how living can be play. In Chapter 7 we sought to overcome the binary opposition of work and play. We saw how they can overlap and intertwine. Mark Twain said: "Work and play are words used to describe the same thing under differing conditions." Speaking of his theory of relativity, Einstein commented: "I thought of that while riding my bicycle." Those people for whom work is a *creative* experience that produces new ideas, art, music, therapy, physics, experimentation, inventions, and innovation are, relatively speaking, a privileged few. In such cases, the seriousness of work (and the cultural imperative to be productive) corresponds with the seriousness of play. It might sound like a contradiction, but taking therapy seriously helps to make it feel like fun (even when therapists swim in an ocean of pain, loss, trauma, and suffering at the same time).

You are often playing more than one role. Consider any important role you play. If parents do not take their role seriously, then parental responsibility is lacking. It is not that everything you do with your kids has to *feel* gravely serious, rather it simply matters, even having fun. Having fun with your kids matters—it is important. Of course, you are not only *playing* a role as a parent; it is also a relationship.

> Fun is a serious matter.

I hardly remember ever having fun with my parents—that is also serious.

> Not having fun is an even more serious matter.

On the other hand, if you feel your role at work or as a parent doesn't matter, it becomes hard to take it seriously, hard to put yourself into it, to care. It isn't enjoyable. You can play around but it isn't *really* fun. The role you play, and the way you play it, makes all the difference. For play to work, to enable finding and creating meaning for yourself in your day-to-day manner of living, play needs to have this serious quality. It needs to mean something more than the merely subjective attitude of those players or observers who populate the arena of play, as Gadamer said.

There is a curious contradiction here: it is necessary to get out of yourself, your preoccupations with yourself, to become yourself, or to live in a more outward-directed and inward-receptive relation to the world. Notice how we shift from a division of self and world to a reciprocal absorption of each in each other. This is the overcoming of a duality. When you are caught up *in* the closed circuit of yourself, then you feel low, your mood drops, things start to feel gloomy, and it becomes hard to see light on the near horizon. There is no way *out* of the closed circuit of your self. It becomes an enclosure. Closed. Foreclosed. Play is shut-down.

The way out of the enclosure of your self comes into view as you get into something or someone else. Opening-up to possibilities for play creates opportunities for closeness.

> Closeness becomes possible, when you open up.

Children tend to play without prompting. Often, though not always, we see children laughing or talking *as if* there were others watching. This may not be that different from a play in the theatre or spectator sport or perhaps also a religious ritual, a more specialised form of play. In each example, an audience is involved. As we said before, play occurs within a closed field. Here closedness allows the game to open. It can open you up, if you let it.

The play occurs in a theatre in which the audience is a part. Here, one of the "walls" that closes in the field of play is opened up. If you imagine a box of four walls, one of the walls is folded down to make a space for the audience in a theatre. In other examples, the spectators surround the field of play that now includes the spectators, audience, or congregation in attendance. Here, play occurs for the others.

The spirit of play for the player is the same as for the spectators, assuming spectators allow themselves to be wholly absorbed in what is being played, as part of it. Shortly after moving to Australia, I attended a football match knowing nothing about Australian Rules Football and not caring either. It was a sociological experiment. I observed Aussies going crazy for their footy, yelling and screaming, swearing abuse at the players when they dropped the ball, going mad when their team won, and so on. I was detached. It all seemed very odd, a group of insane fanatics. Now I am one.

Whether performing a play or participating in it as audience, you must be present to the playing. Presence does not mean viewing from a distance, observing in a detached sense. Presence for the player similarly does not mean going through the motions, pretending, or *playing a role* as make-believe. It means "wholly in it", involved; you are a part of it, and it is a part of you. It matters.

> "To be present means to share."
>
> (Gadamer, 1975, p. 111)

I hadn't thought of "being present" like this before reading Gadamer's quote above. When true sharing occurs in the fullest sense, it has a transcendent quality. You are lifted out of and beyond yourself.

If you are watching a drama in the theatre, then you hope to get into it, to be so absorbed as to be unaware of the theatre, members of the audience, or any other reality than the drama itself. If it is good enough and performed well, then you will feel as if you are living the story and feel all the emotions and dramatic tension of the play *as if* it is your own experience.

You could feel "at one" with the audience sharing this experience but if someone's phone rings—aaarrrgggghhh—then you are jolted out of your absorption in a most irritating way. You are brought back to the reality of being in a theatre audience. You are brought back to your own self-awareness. Have you ever noticed feeling a sense of outrage at the unwanted intrusion of this reality that jolts you out of the drama you are in? This is not sharing.

Sharing is with the actors, the playwright, the director, and everyone involved in mounting the play, and the others watching. When my son and I go to football matches, we are part of the local team. We are playing, too. We are called "members", having joined the club. Even if they are not the best team, we are a part of it. *Proud, Loyal, and Passionate* is our motto. Their victory is our victory. Their loss is our loss. We are in it together.

When we play Scrabble—or, these days, Words with Friends—together on our mobile devices, we might be fiercely competitive, but there is a camaraderie, a kinship, a feeling of family, that we are all racking our brains together to make high-scoring words out of impossible combinations of letters. (Now I enjoy being beaten by my kids.)

> Once, I nearly lost friends from playing Monopoly a little too ferociously. I became fixated on winning and comprehensively destroyed every other player's chances.
>
> In this example, I lost the spirit of play. It became too real, and my ruthlessness was felt as genuine cruelty, also combined with a sort of triumphant attitude at the downfall of my friends' hopes and chances (my *schadenfreude*). I revelled in sadistic pleasure at the pain of their comprehensive defeat.
>
> There was something to be learned here about the nature of play, which is probably why I remember this from so many decades ago. Play can feel like life and death but mustn't become literal murder. That is also not what sharing means. (What's the point if you lose your friends?)

Play and therapy

A singular phenomenon in recent times is the attempt of adult's play to replicate child's play. I am referring to the booming market in so-called "kidult" toys—cuddly toys, Lego, PlayStation, action figures, jigsaws, colouring books, beanie babies, and so on. These toys are not the same as adult toys with "adult content". They are, it seems, an innocent adult-size version of their predecessors—together with adult price tags. The main consumers are Generation Y, although Generation X gets in on the act. It is estimated that this new industry is worth in excess of half a billion dollars and is growing at three times the rate of the whole toy sector.

The usual term for this is "nostalgia"—defined as "a regretful or wistful memory or imagining of an earlier time". This definition (of early twentieth-century coinage) is a soft version of nostalgia, and no doubt most people have experienced it. "Nostalgia" comes from the Greek (*nostos*—home: *algia*—pain), a root that resembles our term "homesickness". Historically, the harder version of "nostalgia" was deemed dangerous enough to cause actual illness and even death, prompting seventeenth-century physicians to diagnose it as a medical disorder, akin to melancholia. Perhaps this harder version echoes in present-day usage. Reputedly, kidult toys recapture "the magic of childhood" and bring out "the big kid in all of us". Fostered by a rosy perspective on childhood (irrespective of the childhood it really was), kidult toys provide pleasure, comfort, irresponsibility, jouissance. Like "fun"—that feel-good concept that saturates advertising—kidult toys are a commodity fetish. They offer adults respite from what Gadamer calls "the actual strain of existence" (1975, p. 94).[71]

I have described the kidult phenomenon to help revisit ideas from earlier sections—the spirit of play, living as play—and so move to the relation between play and therapy. Winnicott says his thesis on this relation is "very simple", it is unequivocal and we revisit it here:

> *Psychotherapy takes place in the overlap of two areas of playing, that of the patient and that of the therapist. Psychotherapy has to do with two people playing together. The corollary of this is that where playing is not possible then the work done by the therapist is directed towards bringing the patient from a state of not being able to play into a state of being able to play.* (1971, p. 38, original emphasis)

I will draw three points from this statement. The first point is straightforward enough. The situation of therapy is a form of *structured* play. As with organised sports and board games, there is a playing area—the consulting room. There are rules of conduct as to what is permissible and what isn't.[72] Huizinga places the play forms in culture in a similar intermediate area of experience, where the consecrated spot of ritual cannot be distinguished from the playground. The arena, the magic circle, the temple, the stage, the court of justice, are all, in form and function, playgrounds within which special rules reign. While the rules in therapy are largely organised around privileging and protecting the client's best interest, there is enough free choice combined with structure to view the interaction as a form of play. If no one follows the rules, the game is over. Chaos erupts. When you play, you play at something—this is the same for children. The game helps define the play. Or the stage frames the space in which a play is performed. The script and its directions help define the set, speech, and action, the characters, and dynamics between them. The score helps define the music, though flourish is allowed. Players are limited within the confines of the game, script, or score, but they have choices.

Playing often delivers a task to its players, something to be aimed for, even mastered. And there is a proper attitude that accompanies play—competing, discovering, slaughtering,

---

[71] Perhaps the surfeit of advertised "fun for sale" highlights the *vacuum* of fun elsewhere—a pervasive feeling that existence is *not*-fun.

[72] R. D. Laing once defined the rules of therapy as "no fucking, no fighting" (personal communication).

building, dominating, creating, subduing, entertaining, all depending on what is being played (including Monopoly). Some professional therapists might resist the idea of equating therapy with play, especially in the context of the extreme suffering of mental illness. Here, it is especially important to remember the *seriousness* of play. We are certainly not playing around. On the contrary, the structure of play, if you can get in the right relation to it, is the ultimate antidepressant and anxiolytic (anxiety-relief medication).

> ## Taking play seriously lightens the strain of existence.

Employing the metaphor of "play" for therapy is a way of looking at it, and not a way of saying what therapy is.

The second point is somewhat more complicated. "Playing together" in "two areas of playing" at first involves a coming-together of two subjective areas of experience—that of the therapist and that of the patient. If sessions continue and playing takes a mature form, then—in the sense of Gadamer's comment quoted in the first section of this chapter—play comes into its own:

> We have seen that play does not have its being in the consciousness of the attitude of the player, but on the contrary, draws the latter into its area and fills him with its spirit. The player experiences the game as a reality that surpasses him. (1975, p. 98)

In this sense, two people in "two areas of playing" participate in the same activity—play as the thing in itself. The patient (no less than the therapist) "achieves self-representation by playing" in a shared game. Whether the spirit of play absorbs the patient and in turn makes them "real"—where self-representation really is representation of an authentic self (the "I am")—depends on the possibility of Winnicott's final remark in the quote above: "*where playing is not possible then the work done by the therapist is directed towards bringing the patient from a state of not being able to play into a state of being able to play*" (1971, p. 38).

This is the third point and, I believe, the most challenging. To those in conditions of the greatest bleakness—the existential vacuum, severe depression and anxiety, dysthymia, and despair—it would be ridiculous to say "All you need to do is play" or "Change your thinking" or "Adjust your attitude and you'll be fine!" On the contrary, in such cases getting into "play" or "playfulness" is the hardest thing. While it's by no means clear how to get *out* of such dark states, being a psychotherapist informs me of two points: (1) you *can* get "better", and (2) it takes work, perseverance, and regular application of yourself (as in regular therapy sessions, often over years). Some of the most deeply depressed, suicidal, and disturbed patients have surprised me by how much improvement can be achieved. The credit goes to the patients for sticking at it when all felt utterly bleak (as you will see in the long case of Luke in Part IV). Credit also belongs to therapists who persevere when loss of faith occurs easily. It occurs more easily for the novice therapist who has not had experience of long, bleak cases that come good in the end. Remembering Aristotle again, part of praxis-for-its-own-sake—in this case, psychotherapy—is the development from positions of novice to excellence to virtuoso, for those who stay the course, apply themselves and hold faith in the process. Those who have done it can testify to its value.[73]

It can be immensely difficult to see your way clear on your own as therapist or patient. Both require support, especially professionally. Consider this: where you are right now (if not already in therapy) is exactly the limit of where you can get to *on your own* to feel better. Another perspective—independent and professional—makes such a difference in this equation. You still have to do the necessary work for yourself, but a professional relationship can become a field of play in which your efforts make a meaningful difference. This is also why proper psychotherapists continue to return to personal therapy and supervision throughout their careers. There is a peculiar paradox when it comes to confronting those ways in which we do not see. To put it in the form of one of R. D. Laing's "knots":

> The range of what we think and do
> is limited by what we fail to notice.
> And because we fail to notice
> *that* we fail to notice
> there is little we can do
> to change
> until we notice
> how failing to notice
> shapes our thoughts and deeds. (Goleman, 1985, p. 24)[74]

It helps to enlist another perspective to notice *that* you failed to notice that you failed to notice. If applied to competitive sport, the meaning of these knotted phrases is easier to grasp. The player fails to notice a problem of technique; failing to do so will not help mend the technique, and the range of the player's accomplishment will correspondingly be limited. Back to tennis coaching, notice how all the professional players continue to be coached even though they are

---

[73] John Heaton told me of a deeply depressed patient of his. This man would beg John to refer him for a lobotomy because his mental state was so unbearable. John refused repeatedly until finally after eleven years of regular therapy, his patient was relieved of his depression. And the relief was lasting. John said he learned more about depression from this patient and his experience of therapy over those years than all the books and his other therapy cases combined.

[74] This quote has been widely attributed to R. D. Laing but originates here with Goleman referring to Laing's book *Knots* (1972). (With thanks to Sidrah Khan for finding this reference when I couldn't.)

better than their coaches. Typically, therapists find a more senior therapist to consult for their own therapy or supervision.

The therapist helps you notice what "you fail to notice" and thus promote your capacity for greater self-awareness. You have to "get into yourself" in order to get out of yourself. Then, you come out of yourself through your absorption in whatever—this is how the game surpasses reality. Therapeutic play requires the therapist to notice how clients find their limits and obstacles in speech and action in the professional relationship. These limits and obstacles are what prevent clients from living a reality beyond those limits. The movement of therapy facilitates the way the client plays in the consulting situation as an analogue for living a reality that surpasses them.

The capacity to achieve improvement or to feel better (Gadamer's "make-believe" goals) is the capacity to be a real player within the reality of therapeutic play—to experience living as meaningful and ultimately creative. In effect, a new sense of self develops that extends into the future. This evokes an image from Gaston Bachelard's book *The Psychoanalysis of Fire* (1964). He often returns to childhood memories, especially to the hearth of his childhood home. Then, the hearth provided delicious warmth, exciting blue-red flames, and fragrance and noises redolent of childhood contentment. More than that, however, the hearth *continued* to play within him, to and fro, to a greater or lesser degree, literally and as a continuing symbol both *in the present*, and as a source of creativity in the future where the hearth-felt thought-kindling produces first a spark and then fire itself, and finally brings thought to boiling point and the creation of thought babies—here thought is alive with meaning-fullness. Bachelard says "like a forgotten fire, a childhood can always flare up again within us" (1964).

Contrast this with what Winnicott calls "fantasying". He gives a long account of a woman patient who, among other things, would spend hours playing the card game patience, also known as solitaire:

> Using what we had done together, I was able to say that patience is a form of fantasying, is a dead end, and cannot be used by me. If on the other hand she is telling me a dream—"I dreamt I was playing patience"—then I could use it and indeed I could make an interpretation. I could say: "You are struggling with God or fate, sometimes winning and sometimes losing, the aim being to control the destinies of four royal families." She was able to follow on from this without help and her comment afterwards was: "I have been playing patience for hours in my empty room and the room really is empty because when I am playing patience I do not exist." (1971, p. 36)

The patient is "playing" but she is dead—"I do not exist". Playing cards by herself is fantasying—a "dead end". I wonder if this applies to others who "play with themselves"?

Fantasying, as we said, is schizoid experience, and its relation to meaninglessness is certainly not confined to therapy but is a cultural phenomenon. There are elements of our present culture in which "playing" is aligned with "magic", and there would seem to be a correlation, at least, between the demise of serious science fiction and the rise of fantasy fiction, films, and computer games in which magic is a *sine qua non*. Magic, too, is a dead end, despite its ability to bounce back as an ageing Harry Potter. All it needs is simply to be *asserted*. How much of this happens in a *sequestered* past or exists in a time and place to which we have no relation, and which bear no fruit. It can still be fun just as fantasying can. The idea of "the magic of childhood" is not the thought of a child or the poetic depictions of a Bachelard. Rather, it is an adult thought which, in the context of kidult nostalgia, is a thought without an heir.

The benefit of therapeutic play is exactly the opposite. It involves the ability to bring *being* into the present so that the "I am" of the patient means *something*. This can be stressful. Participation in therapy can be a precarious experience (for both therapist and patient), involving vulnerability, questions of trust, frustrations, suspicions, silence, and so on. To participate requires a certain attitude nurtured by the therapist, happily appropriating the relation between play and therapy. Funnily enough, when therapy works—much like when living really works—it's magic, but in a very different sense from fantasy or fiction.

* * *

In play, the right-brain functioning of creativity allows a shift from reliance on left-brain cognitions which are primarily rational, analytical, and intellectual.[75] This accounts for the lifting of mood in depression as a benefit of play—this can happen prior to any interpretation of loss that addresses the left brain. Therapy holds the space for right-brain interactions, which also serves attachment functions, reinforcing the central position of relationship in the psychotherapy process. Play + attachment is a formula for change, growth, and development. Attachment also brings a sense of safety to play as the necessary condition of the possibility for creativity and emotional development.[76]

The capacity for play that emerges from therapeutic play does not belong (solely) to the contained enclosure of therapy. It spreads its wings over participation in ordinary living (soulfully). Likewise, therapeutic sharing encompasses those who share ordinary living with you. There are many people—family, friends, those you live with, those you work with, those you play with and socialise with, those you see regularly at the shops, the school, the hospital, the gym, etc.—with whom to share. How do you go about it? There is an interplay. What does it mean to you? Can you get involved with them as people even if only for a brief exchange? Can you remember their names?

When people become a cog in a productivity machine, they may not have issues with meaning—at first. Many people have no difficulty with this, or they have no difficulty for a time

---

[75] See the work of Allan Schore (2012, 2015, 2019), faculty member of the Department of Psychiatry and Biobehavioral Sciences and the UCLA David Geffen School of Medicine, author of a number of volumes on child development.

[76] With thanks to the Developmental Paediatrician Samantha Kaiser for making this point.

and then one day they start to question: *Is this all there is?* Productivity is fine, and necessary to a point. There is nothing wrong with being productive, with making money, with making things, and with building something. Many people seem to be content with the meaning of their life being a matter of making as much money as possible, having as many things as possible, and doing as many things as possible. The themes and discourse of this book, however, point to something beyond this, more *meaningful* than just "playing the game"—in the worst sense.

Many people find they can go along with a role for a time, but then their willingness to do it wears thin and even expires. Your capacity will be limited, and perhaps should be, if you find the activity dehumanising. Sometimes it's worse than that. *I just cannot go into that office for one more day.* The meaningless road is a road well-travelled, but it leads to a dead end. When you feel aggrieved that you are not getting anywhere, you suffer. Reality will not comply with your demand for progress. And you will not surrender to the inevitability of being where you are. It's a standoff. Living becomes characterised by feelings of wretchedness in a game that has become a battle of wills, though life itself has no will at all, it just is.

Whatever it is or is called, life does seem to have a way of playing us. All of us are subject to what happens to us. In this sense, we are thoroughly being played. It is partly for this reason that we need to understand something of the nature and meaning of play—beyond Winnicott—and to participate in it the best way we can. If we are being played, whether we like it or not, whether we have chosen it or not, it is as well to be played in the right spirit.

> Life is a game that plays us.

It is not the hand you are dealt, but how you play it. Of course, some people are dealt a most terrible hand through no fault of their own and it is understandable to feel self-pity or anger or scream protestations of unfairness. There are times when you are called upon to surrender. What follows is a season of adjustment to the way it is. You can fight it, but that tends to make it worse. You can feel that to accept it is to succumb to defeat. Life is not out to win a contest or a war with you.

> If you think life is a battle of wills and you must fight
> against what life throws at you, realise this:
> life has no will, only you do.

Of course, there is no correct way of participating in life any more than there is a fixed way of interpreting it. There is no fixed or correct interpretation in the analysis of a work of art, a piece of theatre, or the performance of a piece of music or dance. The idea of presence as a sharing refers more to a way of participating that gets you out of yourself and into playing with others, as we've been saying.

It is this that gives play a genuinely redemptive function, both in therapy and ordinary living. I am using the word redemptive to mean a restoring of value, of meaning, and of personal investment in the act of playing itself, of playing together, as sharing in living—whatever life throws at you. As such, you become a member of a community, relieved of the pain of isolation (solitaire) and the existential vacuum (monopoly—the monopolisation of wealth). This makes life liveable and able to be lived as a work in process, regardless of what you lack.

Meaning grows out of play as your life plays out.

CHAPTER 12

Play and symbolisation in the professional relationship

> *In psychoanalysis, I believe the most important*
> *question we can ask about psychic phenomena is not*
> *whether they are symbolised in verbal or nonverbal terms,*
> *or even whether they are conscious or unconscious,*
> *but instead whether they are* **meaningful**.
> Donnel B. Stern (2019, p. 21, original emphasis)

For Stern, following the quote above, what is meaningful emerges from unformulated experience—his theory of the unconscious—as well as verbal reflections, both being formed into linguistic expressions as a function of the interpersonal professional relationship.

Across the mental health disciplines, there are varying degrees of awareness of how important the professional relationship is. Often, it is the factor that stands out as making the most difference in what patients say has helped them. Yet, the connection between patient and therapist is difficult to research. There have been many studies and as I understand it, the research on therapy regularly reaches the conclusion that the relationship accounts for much more variance in outcome than the "brand" of therapy.[77] It would be difficult to pin down the value of the professional relationship because of many intangible elements. However, there is now significant empirical evidence confirming *the therapeutic alliance influences outcome across a range of psychotherapies, despite their therapeutic and technical differences*. One study went further in concluding that the professional relationship also positively influenced the effectiveness of both medication and placebo.

---

[77] With thanks to Nancy McWilliams for making this point (and countering my bias against research).

What this finding suggests is that the therapeutic alliance may strongly influence the placebo response embedded in pharmacotherapy as a nonspecific factor above and beyond the specific pharmacologic action of the drug. The therapeutic alliance may help to create a "holding" environment in which the acceptance of taking a drug may be enhanced and permit concerns to be addressed and worked through within the context of a supportive and collaborative relationship (such as fears of dependence on medication, resistance, and demoralisation regarding the delayed or variable effects of medication or placebo and the difficulty tolerating the discomforts of drug side effects). (Krupnick et al., 1996)

There is the client and the therapist, two entities, two people. Then there is the bond, the connection, the rapport between them, a third entity (that is also not an entity because it isn't a "thing"). There is a physical reality or presence of the two people but what is between them is not physical, it is metaphysical. It is sometimes referred to as "the working alliance" in the literature. In psychoanalysis, it is the transference/countertransference relationship. In academic and clinical psychology, formerly psychologists were supposed to maintain a professional distance and separateness. They were trained not to get too involved. Due to a growing evidence base confirming the centrality of the professional relationship, there is now wider recognition of its importance for therapeutic effectiveness. The American Psychological Association even released a statement of policy adopting a resolution on the Recognition of Psychotherapy Effectiveness (2012) that begins:

psychotherapy is rooted in and enhanced by a therapeutic alliance between therapist and client/patient that involves a bond between them ... (The American Psychological Association, 2012)

In developmental psychotherapy, the relationship *is* the therapy.

A personal bond cannot be seen by an objective look because it is not an object. Yet, it is one of the most important qualities—if not the most important quality—of therapy and its effectiveness. A relationship—any relationship—is not a singular or fixed thing. It is always unfolding, changing; it is more like a living organism. As I said before, it is difficult to even talk about mental health practices because each practice—psychology, psychiatry, psychotherapy—is not one unified "thing". Each is personal and interpersonal, even when the professional is keeping separate and formal.

Any discussion of meaning, where it comes from and how it is created, has everything to do with relationship. It might refer to your relationship with your loved ones, your work, sport, creative pursuits, religion, political causes, or whatever matters, as we've been saying. Meaning waxes and wanes and is also like a living organism. It comes to life and grows through the play of symbolisation.

Symbolisation and play have a natural relationship, they go together, even belong together. Each enhances the other, they bring out the best in each other, they were made for each other. Symbolisation gives play meaning and play enables symbolisation to flourish. I want to consider play and symbolisation and the relation between them, and their relation to the professional relationship in the following clinical examples.

Jane

I see Jane for her first session, and in a flash of clarity, I make an interpretation—"You feel misunderstood by your partner, so you push her away, you create distance, then you feel resentful at the lack of connection"—and I think to myself *yes, that was on the mark but I'm not sure it meant much to her*. Two years later, after many more instances of the above theme have been discussed, I say "You feel misunderstood by your partner, so you push her away, you create distance, then you feel resentful at the lack of connection". This time it appears to be a light-bulb moment, an awakening, a revelation—the accompanying feeling gives a sense of *You cannot carry on like that any longer because you keep suffering the effects of this pattern. Enough!* Jane then goes and explains to her partner the reasons for this feeling of being misunderstood. The partner "gets it" and Jane feels closer and more connected, opposite to how it has been.

I made the same communication as I did in the first session, verbatim. It was an identical interpretation at an identical juncture, as my client reported much the same dynamic two years on. Two years later, my words have a weight, substance, *meaning* that was not registered in the first session. How could it? We had only just met. It's not *just* the words but the words in the context of a professional relationship that makes the difference. Meaning is context-dependent as well as content-dependent. It is great to be right, but that is not all there is to it, and not all there is to what makes therapy work.

Who I am, the speaker, is a "different person" after two years of regular sessions. I'm not a *different person*, rather, I am a different person to Jane. Jane is a different person to me. I know her whereas I didn't know her before. She knows me, in my professional being. So, the "same" interpretation is not the same. It means something radically different (to her) though the same words were said, and the same meaning intended.

In a further example of this scenario, Jane "acts out", misses a session without warning, is late for the next one, and arrives with a cold and distant expression on her face, she looks uninterested in speaking to me and feels remote.

I say: What's going on?

Jane: I didn't really want to come today, I just wasn't in the mood, and I don't have anything to talk about. Everything's fine, really.

Me: I'm glad to hear everything's fine but you didn't attend your last appointment. In the past you have always let me know if you couldn't make it.

Jane: Yes, I know, I was so busy, there was so much going on. [*Sounds vague*]

Me: In our last session, I said I thought you were angry with your mother about something she said to you and you had quite a reaction, you thought I got it wrong and you weren't angry with her at all. In fact, you said you thought your mother was right.

Jane: Yes, I remember that. I really didn't like hearing the way you put it. I was angry about what my mother said but not angry at her. I was angry because she was right!

Me: So, could this be an example of you pushing me away, creating distance when I didn't understand you—this is something we know has been a tendency—and then you wind up resentful at the disconnect. I felt you were quite far away when we started today.

Jane: [*Thinking about it*]

Me: [*Continuing*] Are you aware of feeling any resentment toward me? I wonder if it means something that you missed last session, didn't contact me, and arrived late for this one?

Jane: I see, you think I am 'speaking" through my actions, expressing a feeling …

Me: What do you think?

This is an example of not-knowing as a professional expert—I put my view tentatively—and an example of the use of a professional relationship to analyse transference. It is also an example of the symbolic order of language being brought into the relationship between us, as I see Jane's actions as saying and meaning something. I invite her to consider if she was expressing something indirectly, and without words, because saying it brings that meaning and corresponding feelings between us *to* the relationship, whereas acting out takes the meaning *out* of it. We, all of us, speak all the time through our actions, also by how we look, our way of moving, gesticulating, and everything that is expressive in our way of being. Symbolisation involves putting this into words—articulating sense and meaning to the feelings and actions that constitute our relationships.

Not everything can be put into words—or should be. Sometimes, it is preferable, and indeed a stronger communication, to act directly than to put it into words. And sometimes, there simply are no words. When we reach the limit of language, it is best to remain silent.

> "Whereof one cannot speak, thereof one must be silent."
> (Ludwig Wittgenstein)

Richard

A client, Richard, tells me that he finds it hard to show love for his son. He does love him, he loves him beyond measure, but cannot show it. His son has endured emotional deprivation, Richard said, throughout his childhood. He wants to be a better father and doesn't agree with this way of being. He knows why he's like this but cannot change it.

Richard's father was like this except worse. His father believed in being hard on him, harsh and critical, to make him a better man than himself. It didn't, and Richard hated being treated like this as both child and adult. But the word "father" means being like that.

As a father to his son, he has become like his father to him as a child. This is also called "an identification". The idea of symbolisation directs our focus upon the meaning of the word *father* to Richard. It is not just the meaning of the *word* but the meaning of his way of being a father, *fathering*.[78]

The task of therapy is to crack open the meaning of the word *father* so that its meaning isn't foreclosed or limited to my client's own experience of being *fathered* in this self-same way. Subjection to language can be a prison or a source of freedom. Fathering doesn't have to be like *your* father or your experience of being fathered.

Interestingly, Richard told me that when he saw me for the first time, he was overwhelmed by anxiety because my white beard reminded him of his father. He felt desperately afraid that I would treat him as his father had. My being a different race, colour, size, age, and ethnicity did not alter this apprehension. The white beard was enough to evoke the association.

When I turned out to be kind and supportive, it was disorientating, indeed even disillusioning. I am older than Richard, not that much actually, but that also doesn't alter the point that Richard felt *as if* he were having a positive experience of *fathering* from me, even though we both know that I am not his father nor trying to be. I am genuinely fond of him, and he can feel that. Therapy is not re-parenting, yet there are new experiences to be had *as if* with a parent.

While I can point out how his concept of *father* has kept him at a cool distance from his son—and this is worth saying—I suspect his experience of our relationship will make more of a difference than all the interpretations under the sun. I can't prove this or do research on it to produce *evidence*, this is the kind of knowledge that clinical experience generates. Practice-based evidence is subjective but that doesn't mean it isn't true or of value. The subjective can also be objectively correct, though still a form of interpretation.

Alice

A forty-four-year-old client, Alice, tells me a dream:

> After an event at work, I dreamt I was in a house (I didn't recognise it). It was a Federation-style house with a large, wooden veranda all around it. It was covered with my childhood toys. What were they doing there? I wondered. I started to pick them up, but I didn't know where to put them. Then I woke up. What do you think it means?

---

[78] In this example, the meanings of identification, a psychological defence in its psychoanalytic usage and symbolisation in my usage, are much the same. One difference is context. Symbolisation, like focusing binoculars, references my client's use of language and crystallises its effect upon him. I prefer the construction: "he is subject to the symbolic order" over "he defends himself against emotional vulnerability through the defense of identification". Notice how the second construction presupposes agency. Yet, my client says he cannot help it or change this.

Me: Do you have any ideas?

Alice: I had the idea that these are relics from my childhood that need to be overcome for me to develop as an adult. [*I think she knows I am into ideas of development*]

Me: It reminds me of how you played on your own as a child. You have two brothers, but they are so much older than you and so they did their own things most of the time.

Alice: Yes [*looking interested*], go on,

Me: Maybe the toys are there for you to play with?

Alice: I don't really know how to play.

Me: It helps to have someone to play with.

Alice: I never did.

[*We discussed the toys, what they looked like, what sort of toys were there, etc.*]

Alice: How can I learn to play at this stage?

Me: We are playing with the images of your dream, their possible meanings, and the questions arising from them, right now.

Here, I am trying to draw Alice's attention to the connection between us and the quality of play in our interaction, something that is elusive to her, as she had little experience of either connection or play as a child. In terms of symbolisation, we are opening possible meanings of *play* which is where our discussion of her dream has taken us. For Alice, "play" has become something of a dead metaphor. She thinks she needs to put the toys away, as something to be overcome. I think they need to stay out for her to get involved with them. She doesn't know how. I want to bring the metaphor of play to life, by opening up different possibilities, different ways of playing with the meaning of play in the context of our professional relationship. I can have a different view without *imposing* mine upon her.

There can be a quality, a sense of play in so much of what you do or think. Indeed, you will feel lighter for the benefit of this.

Judy and Sean

Judy is a client doing a Master of Science degree course in Clinical Psychology. She brought up her case of an eleven-year-old boy, Sean, following a distressing session of family therapy. In the session, everyone in Sean's family had pointed their finger at him as being "the problem"; he was difficult and forever causing strife. Sean became more and more withdrawn until he was unreachable. Judy shut it down, suspended the session, to protect Sean from further persecution. She took Sean into a private room. She tried to talk with him about how he felt about what was happening with his family, being blamed, being identified as "the problem" and the associated emotions—resentment, anger, and disappointment—from his family members. Sean didn't want to talk.

They sat in a kind of tense and awkward silence interspersed with a few gentle questions from her. He wouldn't engage. Then she asked "Is there anything I can do for you right now? Anything you would like?" With no hesitation at all Sean said, "Can we play that game you showed me last time I was here?" It was a word game, making words out of a jumble of letters. "Yes, of course." Judy was delighted to oblige. "Sure, no problem." She deliberately combined letters that made potential words of relevance to what was happening such as *brother, anger, unfairness, blame, conflict, and family.* As soon as they started playing, the tension and awkwardness disappeared, and Sean was able to talk, happy to answer her questions, open to addressing issues connected with the words of the game and willing to discuss the issues with his family.

Play enabled therapy, as words could become symbolised, and meanings emerge through playing the word game together. As play, considering what his experience means is easy and agreeable. Sean doesn't want "clinical psychology", "family therapy", "psychotherapy", "development", "medication", or "treatment"—he wants someone to play with, who wants to play with him. Then they can talk about anything.

I like this example because it shows how play and symbolisation go well together and how the therapy emerges out of this combination in the context of a professional relationship. It doesn't matter to me what the professional identification is—psychologist, psychotherapist, psychiatrist, counsellor, mental health nurse, social worker, doctor; it matters what a mental health professional *does*. Here, Judy, a trainee, made her young patient feel safe. She protected him, showed care, accommodated his wish to play a word game, and created a rapport that helped Sean open up and have a meaningful discussion with her.

Sarah and Ted

Sarah and Ted are attending a couple's therapy session. She doesn't like him pressuring her for sex and regarding her disinterest as a symptom of a disorder, she said.

Ted to Sarah:	You're so cold, you always seem busy with other things, preoccupied, and distracted when it comes to sex or if there is an opportunity. You'd rather look at your phone. [*!*]
Sarah to me:	I feel more turned-off by these negative comments, as if he is some kind of expert on how I should feel, or when I should want sex with him.
Me to Ted:	Your focus is critical of Sarah, which is a long way from foreplay if you are seeking to warm her up to the possibility of being sexual with you. It sounds like you are pathologising her rather than expressing how you are feeling [*symbolising*] such as: I am feeling sexually frustrated or I'm about to go away for two weeks and I'm afraid if we don't make love, it will be a long time before there is any chance of it.

Symbolising how you feel in words is a positive alternative to taking pot shots, aggressive jabs, poking critiques, and nasty asides to your *beloved* partner. Also, notice the word *play* in foreplay.

Ted took in what I was saying. He had initiated these sessions because Sarah was beginning to make references to leaving, to ending their twenty-four-year marriage, to going separate ways, and "calling it a day". He was desperately afraid of losing her. The urgency of his situation made my communications carry more weight. He was determined to listen and do things differently. He put great stock in our professional relationship even though we had only just met. He and Sarah were bordering on crisis, so he listened and started to treat her differently. It made a huge difference to her. She stopped wanting to leave and started wanting to make love with him more often, though it would probably never be as much as he would like.

When he put how he was feeling into a direct expression to her, she could feel sympathy and also empathy for him, and it made her feel more open to connecting with him. That meant something to her, instead of her having to defend herself from the threat of being made "bad or wrong" for how she felt or what she didn't feel. She was free to feel whatever she did feel and to express herself accordingly. The freedom to symbolise opened possibilities between them. This, in turn, lightened the tension and the feeling of pointing in different directions, wanting different things, not being on the same page. Sexuality, expressed as the play of foreplay (rather than crude comments like *are you up for it?*) becomes sexier, brings a feeling of *eros*, and stimulates sexual desire and arousal, so important for healthy relationships, especially longer-term ones, to stay alive.

Play gives the sexuality of this couple a quality of freshness and even fun, rather than a stale negotiation. It can mean something without having to be symbolised in words. The giving of physical affection without agenda, no strings attached, says more than a dry communication in words. Symbolisation is a way of referring to expressiveness and not restricted to verbal communications in words. The popular book *The 5 Love Languages* (Chapman, 1992) comes to mind: words of affirmation, also touch, spending time, giving, and acts of service—the latter four are "languages" not based on verbal expression.

Amanda and her psychiatry registrar therapist

I supervise a psychiatry registrar[79] on the psychotherapy of his very first case of "long-term therapy" (forty sessions is long-term in psychiatry, it's short-term to me). Amanda is a young mum with a baby that she has brought along with her to her third session. She couldn't arrange childcare, she said. About halfway into the session, without warning, she hands her therapist, the registrar, her baby to hold while she rifles around in her bag for her phone. She's taken some notes that she wants to retrieve for the session, she switches on the phone, waits for it to start up, finds her notes, reads them through before continuing.

---

[79] Registrar is the term for a psychiatry trainee in Australia and the UK but in the United States the term is "resident".

The psychiatry registrar was feeling worried that normally holding babies for patients isn't part of his role and was it okay? I said I wasn't overly worried about whether he broke any rules, I was more interested in what it might mean.

Me: What do you think it means that Amanda handed you her baby to hold?
Him: I don't know, I was so worried about whether it was okay, I didn't think about that.
Me: Could it be that Amanda was "saying" she trusts you to hold the baby part of herself, that she can bring this into the therapy process with you, even while she gets on with other adult things like being a mum herself?

Handing him the baby could be called a pre-symbolic communication, as it is symbolised not in words but in action. It is important to translate and understand what actions mean, while at the same time recognising that my interpretation here is not the only possibility, not necessarily correct, or the best way of reading the meaning of Amanda's action. This is why therapy seeks to open up possibilities of meaning and bring them into the conversation between us. Often, you know when a meaning is right because you feel it in your body. Conversely, your body's lack of reaction may signal that it does not feel right. When that is the case, often the meaning is not right or not complete. Sometimes it is right but not the right time. Coming to what something means is a process I call the embodiment of symbolisation.

I offer my perspective in a deliberately indefinite way *Could it be …* Yes, it could be, but it doesn't have to be. I don't want to impose my idea dogmatically, rigidly, or fuel a dynamic where the registrar knows nothing, and I know everything (the professional expert). You can elicit idealisation, but the registrar won't learn much, and is likely to feel empty. I don't want to make supervisees feel empty any more than I want to make clients feel that way. If we can play with different ideas, different ways of looking at things, different possible meanings, then we develop capacities for improvisation that can be brought to other clinical moments. This improvisational mode works better than when a professional expert imposes a pre-determined perspective derived from some external source such as a research study or a treatment manual constructed by academics with scant clinical experience. It is the difference between personal and impersonal, and between a dominance/submissive relationship and a relationship in which each party's view is worthy of consideration.

Developmental psychotherapy, as I argue here, is more about play, meaning, and relationship—pointing in quite a different direction from the medical model or the scientist practitioner model of psychology. Are they compatible? Some psychiatrists are exclusively biological—it seems to be a matter of personal preference. Can we do both? Some psychologists have started calling themselves "psychotherapists", though they haven't been trained in psychotherapy. It is hard to see how the treatment of mental illness can point in two opposing directions at once and still hope to be effective. Many mental health professionals seem to be making it up as they go along; I hear about it in the clinic when they come for supervision. This might sound equally improvisational, but that is not what I mean. The Developmental

Psychotherapist improvises within a well-established process and structure of therapy, pre-scribed throughout this book and many others. Not-knowing does not mean *I don't have a clue!*

Thomas Szasz was right when he said "define or be defined" (1990, p. 55).[80]

Lois (a longer example)

I asked a client, Lois, how she felt about becoming a "couple" with Spencer, the man she's been seeing for over a year. Lois replied: "I can't know how I feel until I know that I matter to him." I was struck by the immediacy of her response without even a moment to consider the question.

Here is the background: over the past weekend, Spencer had told Lois about his travel plans for next year. In each case, whether he planned to travel near or far, she was not included. He spoke thus: "I'm going there" and then in April "I'm going there" and in June "I'm going some-where else" and in October "I have to go to this place for work". They were *his* travel plans, not *theirs*. He was planning to make these trips as a separate, individual person and wasn't thinking they might go together, or even to offer her the option of travelling with him. She noticed. This made her feel that she didn't matter, indeed couldn't matter much to him and that he didn't really see them as a couple. That impression was contradicted by other communications in which he had referred to her as his girlfriend or partner.

After this happened, that same night, she had a dream:

> I had a list of all the places in the world I'd like to go to with Spencer, but I couldn't read the names of any of them.

The absence of "her" in his travel plans is a symbolic lack, it gives expression to something missing. If she doesn't exist in his plans, how can they be a couple? It is the presence of an absence. The absence of symbolisation of them as a couple means something, it *says* they are "not a couple" in his mind in the context of his plans. The not-saying says something. She felt hurt and confused, though it took her a little while to put it all together and realise why.

The dream gives a similar sense. If we don't take it literally, there is a sense that she would like to "go somewhere" with Spencer, perhaps many "places"—here "places" is a metaphor for union, for a togetherness, closeness, for travelling as a couple to a "place" of love. It is not that specific, but this is the point. She cannot know how she feels about being a couple until she feels that she matters—it makes so much sense. The "places" on the list in her dream cannot be read, cannot be symbolised. Yet.

In the next session, Lois told me that Spencer admitted to her that he wished he could get back with his ex-wife even though she had treated him "monstrously". This was insult upon

---

[80] The quote in full is "In the animal kingdom, the rule is: eat or be eaten; in the human kingdom: define or be defined" (1990, p. 55).

injury, though Spencer did acknowledge that both his remarks about travelling plans and this admission were hurtful.

Lois started to feel angry, then anger gave way to tears and as she started to cry, she said to Spencer: "You really hurt me and that's not okay."

Her whole body started to shake, she trembled, hyperventilated, felt rising panic, and then couldn't breathe. Spencer held her. More importantly, he held the space, the tension of emotion without trying to fix it or make her feel better. He stayed with her in the discomfort zone, he stayed connected. He said "It's okay to feel like that." In saying so, she could feel genuine care, and her tense state gave way to deep sobs. Something was being released with all the snotty, guttural, spasmodic, and convulsive shaking that went with it. These were the deep sobs of feelings buried from her childhood, of dynamics in which she was not allowed to have emotional needs or express her feelings, especially if hurt or needy; at the same time, they were also the sobs of hurt from the present relationship. Past and present reverberated like an echo chamber, inflating emotional pain and then release.

The release of a deep historic trauma felt relieving and freeing. Then they had passionate sex. She wanted to, and it made her feel better.

This is an example of embodied symbolisation. It involves words—saying how hurt she felt—but words that are also grounded in the felt-experience of the body, with simultaneous reference to both past and present experience. Her embodied symbolisation was released by his care. Even though he was the source of emotional injury, he was still with her, in a connected and genuine way. She knew that she did matter to him and could also feel this through their sexual intimacy.

She could feel what was possible between them without getting bogged in judgements as to whether it is enough or not enough, definitions of whether they are a couple or not, and needing to know where this is going, ultimately.

After that experience, she reported a series of dreams:

1. She was negotiating to have a sexual foursome with another couple. *Really*, she wanted to have sex with the man—not sure who—but she had to include her partner and the man's partner to make that happen.
   (She couldn't remember the details of most of these dreams.)
2. She was discussing how to stop sexual abuse from happening; the way she was advocating this was by having sexual threesomes.
3. Here, there was a snippet of a dream in which she was trying to map the best way to protect everyone from the possibility of sexual abuse.
4. This dream happened the night before the morning of her session: she had done something (the implication was something wrong, perhaps criminal) and there was an image of her being put into a car with four men. They penetrated her sexually in *every imaginable way* with objects, and parts of their own bodies. It was horrible—like porno—then the dream changes. The next part involves an old friend of hers, Jade, an activist against sexual abuse—there were beggars around—Lois

was muttering about her alter-ego called Mr Doubtful. Then she is with a different friend in New York with two little kids and fireworks were about to be set-off.

Lois wanted to know what I thought of the dreams.

Me: I notice a confusion between having sex with multiple partners as if to prevent sexual abuse.

Lois: My mother had taught me from a young age that sex was a trading card, a bargaining chip, it was what men wanted and had to be given if you were ever to expect to get anything from them such as what you really want which is to be looked after in both emotional and practical ways. "If you don't put out sexually then you won't get what you want or need."

Me: In the dreams, I'm missing love or even a sense of the erotic for you. Sex is employed for a purpose—a trading card—to achieve a particular aim or goal.

Lois: Yes, there is no sense of sex as a loving transaction between two people.

Me: Transaction?

Lois: Yes [*catching herself at the same time*], I realise I used the word "transaction" which makes it sound like commerce.

At the end there was a sense of a thirty-six-year-old woman discovering an aspect of her own sexuality, that it didn't have to be something to be used to procure favour from a man. The references to sexual abuse were also echoes of incidents at age five and later as a teenager. These had been remembered and discussed, but here there was a curious contradiction. It was as if she felt she had to be sexual to prevent abuse. There was also a sense that sex devoid of love, or even sexual arousal for its own sake, can feel abusive, like an exploitation, if it is a corruption of what sex can mean.[81]

At the end, there was an important moment where the meaning of "transaction" strikes both of us at once. We both register that in symbolising sex in that way, it means something, something revealing and questionable at once. This is exactly what needs to be called into question, to open the possibility for sex to be experienced more lovingly, and more erotically (I like Ester Perel's term "erotic intensity" (2007)) to change the meaning of the word (and so, the act) from what it has meant before now. This also points to what I mean by development, for her sexuality to be more freely experienced without having to involve a transaction, an agenda—trying to get something else she wants or needs—and to it becoming an expression of how she feels sexually, what she wants (or doesn't), and what exists between her and her partner.

Maybe for her to develop a capacity for erotic intensity as an expression of love and desire, without having to purchase anything from him in return, would make a difference to how Spencer sees the possibility of being a couple with Lois, and to "travelling" together?

---

[81] I hasten to add *nothing against meaningless sex* if that is what you both want, as consenting adults.

Cindy and Tammy

Cindy and Tammy had lived together for seven years until Tammy moved out and called off the relationship much to Cindy's dismay. A few months later Cindy consulted me to help her make the transition from being in a couple to being single. She was quite down-to-earth, practical, efficient, business-like—she was in pain but getting on with her life. She had many friends.

By her account, Tammy was an astrologer, Tarot-card reader, she was a bit hippie, someone who floated around, attractive, oozed sexuality, full of flirtation, and a free spirit. Cindy had supported Tammy financially for most of their relationship and Tammy had no hesitation in asking people for help. She didn't have her own home, not even a rental; Tammy did house-sitting, and went from one often posh home to the next. She had many contacts, and there always seemed to be someone who wanted their garden tended or pets or property looked after while they were away. Some people even paid her for this service. Reverse rent.

Tammy had a three-night gap between house-sits and had nowhere to go. She could sleep in her car but didn't want to. She could crash at a friend's place, but that was far away. So, she asked Cindy if she would put her up for the three nights.

Cindy was quite taken aback. She had been putting her energy into separating, into "getting over" the relationship with Tammy and had suffered seeing her having fun on social media. It was not what Cindy needed at all. Cindy was a generous and caring person, and on reflection, she thought she could cope and help her ex even if it would be a little uncomfortable. That is what she did.

From a position of greater separateness, she observed how Tammy did not offer to reciprocate despite frequent opportunities. Cindy made Tammy breakfast when Tammy could just as easily have offered to make Cindy breakfast. When Cindy drove her to collect her things and had to put fuel in the car, Tammy could have offered a contribution, but chose not to. When they stopped off at the grocery store, Tammy suggested they buy some expensive charcuterie but stood back when it came time to pay for it. And when there was clearing up that needed to be done, Tammy was tired or had to make a phone call. Cindy became increasingly aware of how one-sided her relationship had been for most of the time they were together. Here it was in stark relief: they're not together, but Tammy still feels entitled to being looked after.

The three nights passed without incident. It was okay. Tammy didn't say much of a thank you, there was no card, no acknowledgement until Cindy received a text message that said "You are a beautiful person and you provided such a loving and healing space for me".

In the moment of receiving it, Cindy had an insight: for Tammy, her warmth, affection, and affirmations were a form of currency. Cindy saw that Tammy believed that what she gave at a personal level was a fair, if not generous, exchange for what she received at a material level. It hadn't really been a particularly loving or healing space. In fact, to protect herself and preserve her emerging separateness, Cindy was reserved and contained. She didn't want to let Tammy back into her heart. She had already worked at moving on. Now, she could see the former customary feeling of being used for what it was, what it meant.

> You feel it when you're in it,
> but you can't see it,
> until you're out of it.

Here, the symbolisation of "You are a beautiful person providing a loving and healing space" had a gratuitous, false quality, as if to provide some element of compensation. It was like giving someone a gift that you like but they don't. Cindy registered this clearly. Though the words *appeared* to be from the heart, they didn't ring true. I would call this a disembodied symbolisation. If anything, Cindy was reminded of how often she had felt used more than loved. She recognised that Tammy had stayed together with her for a long time, well after the intimacy of their relationship had expired. She embraced the experience of Tammy staying over three nights as confirmation that she was better off out of this relationship, even though it hadn't been her choice to separate.

Formless, unintegrated experience

In playing, adults, like children, are free to be creative, both in therapy and in their lives.

> It is in playing and only in playing that the individual child or adult is able to be creative and to use the whole personality, and it is only in being creative that the individual discovers the self. (Winnicott, 1971, p. 54)

But how do we get to *a whole personality?* It is a product of integration but sometimes unintegration needs to happen first.

> It is only here, in this unintegrated state of the personality, that that which we describe as creative can appear. This if reflected back, *but only if reflected back*, becomes part of the organized individual personality, and eventually this in summation makes the individual to be, to be found; and eventually enables himself or herself to postulate the existence of the self. (Winnicott, 1971, p. 64, original emphasis)

To reach for the creativity of play and symbolisation in the professional relationship, sometimes personalities need to come apart in order to come together in a better order.

In formless, unintegrated experiencing, anything goes. Children are likely to make a mess, things don't make sense, and order and structure are nowhere to be found. For carers, this is uncomfortable—should it be allowed? There are great opportunities for creativity and development. For children, it is not a matter of letting them go feral, allowing them to run wild, and encouraging dysregulation. Rather, carers must *reflect back* the child's own creations even if messy and out-of-order; that is, out of an order that is familiar and comfortable. The same principle applies to therapists and their patients when the usual psychological structures dis-integrate.

When patients let go of their integration, it can be frightening for therapists. It can seem like the wrong direction, as therapy is so often working *towards* integration. We may have to go backward (in regression) to go forward (towards integration)—that is, part of a developmental process.

Therapists, like the carers of young children, reflect back, validate, and give understanding to formless, unintegrated experience—that gives it value.

> Sometimes, you go backwards to go forwards.
> Then, regress becomes progress.

This is not simply a small matter of a pleasant developmental moment called play. Winnicott is proposing play as the basis of *the whole of our experiential existence*. Emotional development is not simply a linear progression from a position of relative lesser development to a position of greater, more integrated sense of self. Rather, development proceeds in two different directions at once. For greater integration to be possible, there needs to be a capacity for formless experience, for regression, for disorder, even chaos, perhaps experienced as nonsense. Again, this is messy. The other, tidier direction of coming-together, growing more responsible and mature, is more comfortable. What if this part of development also requires evolving towards a greater capacity for a relaxing of being *together* (in yourself), for letting it all go, and not having to be oh-so-responsible, and for play? Throw the toys and make a mess (like children). This also includes making a mental mess, allowing your mind to roam free, to space out, to go to pieces without undue fear of not being able to function, never coming together again. Many people take psychotropic recreational drugs to reach to such states. Sometimes, people feel the need to force themselves into an unintegrated state, knowing there is something of value there, if they are unable to "get there" otherwise. On this note, more and more people have difficulties sleeping, a "natural" unintegrated state.

There is a driving need to reach to unintegrated experience and, at the same time, not enough space in ordinary living to allow it, even through a night's sleep. Now, many people cannot sleep or sleep enough, without forcing sleep through meds, weed, alcohol, exercise, sex, *or something*—often a combination. One couple referred to manually giving each other an orgasm as "a sleeping pill". They weren't making love; they were taking tension out of their respective systems. Tension is felt physically and also in the form of busy mental activity.

Dismantling your own mental operations can lead to formless, unintegrated experience. Sometimes, your customary manner of being and doing—the pattern of your thought and actions once established—benefits from being taken apart. The reversion to formless experience opens possibilities of coming together in a better order. This example shows the value of regression to a less-formed state in the context of a developmental psychotherapy process and professional relationship.

Damien was a thirty-two-year-old who came for therapy in a terrible state. Sometimes, he couch-surfed or slept rough, outside, wherever he might land for the night. He abused every drug he could get. He abused alcohol (a lot). He spent every cent he could get his hands on. He ate the cheapest junk-food. And chased women for sex. He was good looking and had no trouble, but it was never enough. He was never satisfied. He didn't like himself—that puts it mildly—and he didn't really like anyone else. He could see his pattern of living was a disaster. He came seeking radical change.

It was clear to both of us that his pattern of living was a direct reflection of sedimented patterns of thinking. He had a hostile relation to himself and to the world (somewhat reminiscent of Clarissa from Chapter 3). Living was a form of combat, and the aim was survival while avoiding his own inner life (mental state).

After two years of therapy, Damien regressed to an earlier stage of development. Sometimes, he seemed two years old. He would curl up in his chair and cry, sometimes for the whole session. It was quite a sight as he was six feet, six inches tall and strongly built. Here was a huge, muscular man before me, yet all I could see was a baby. He was broken-down and felt broken, he was profoundly sad and child-like—session after session.

Eventually, he moved to a less regressed but still young position that seemed more like an adolescent than a young child. Here, Damien was angry. He wasn't angry *at* me, more at the hand life dealt him. There was strength in anger. He would pound the arm of his chair and sometimes punch the brick wall next to him. I felt afraid he'd hurt himself (or break the wall) but I never feared his violence. He wasn't like that. If anything, I felt he was grateful for my willingness to baby-sit him.

With time, the dis-integration of his former mental structures were re-forming into something stronger, with a greater capacity to suffer frustration. He was growing up. The more he grew up, the more he was able to symbolise in an adult way; his speech reflected his emerging maturation.

Then, Damien decided to put energy into work. He got a job, part-time at first, as a maintenance man. It wasn't well-paid; he was pushed around, exploited, but he put up with it. At least he was earning a bit of money and lived within a more structured frame. He learned and grew more skilled. Fast forward a few years: Damien went on to start his own maintenance company. It serviced large organisations such as shopping complexes, office blocks, and government buildings.

The more successful he was, the better he felt. The better he felt, the harder he worked. He gave up drugs and alcohol completely along the way. And he fell in love with a beautiful woman, went on to marry and have a child together.

Some years after therapy finished, they invited me to their home to introduce me to their baby. I was amazed because their home was nicer than mine and fully paid-off! Damien was brimming with pride. Envy aside, I was thrilled with these developments for him. He had designed and renovated the property himself, in his spare time. He was showing-off. Fair enough—he'd come such a long way.

Therapy had involved six years of weekly sessions, and twice-weekly when regressed. Damien had gone through an experience of unravelling his personal psychology and re-forming it in a better order—through his regression.

I had never really seen much evidence of Damien's being able to play until I saw him at his home with his baby daughter, bouncing her around, down on the ground with toys, singing her songs, reading her books—and in this mode, he was happy in a way I had never seen in sessions. A life worth living.[82]

What if we are losing the (potential) value of mental "disorders" by treating, curing, or medicating them out of existence? Although I don't think this applies to every disorder, it could apply to some.

Formless experience for adults happens in different ways, of which regression is one. Some people use substances, and some are better than others—MDMA, Ayahuasca, mushrooms, ketamine, cannabis, trips—I will leave the legality to you as it varies. There are movements to do research and maximise the potential therapeutic benefits of such substances legally.[83] However you get there, my principal point is that formless, unintegrated experience can have therapeutic benefits and result in developmental growth.

*   *   *

Winnicott's idea that play occurs in the continuum of time and space raises questions for me. In one way of looking at it, the very experience of time and space is itself probably a function of the capacity for play. Time and space are fixed entities—we can measure each—but the way they are experienced is not fixed.

Experientially, time can be an eternity or can flash by in the blink of an eye. Space can feel expansive and open, or a room can feel like a shoebox. Time can drag when we are bored to death. The space of one's body can be light as a feather or a lead weight, or a dead weight.

---

[82] Sounds perfect but Damien and his wife also had some terrible times too, tumultuous and disturbing. They worked hard at resolving things and not separating. They are expecting their second child and are doing better than they were (as of 2021).

[83] For example, see https://mindmedicineaustralia.org/ in Australia.

Different clients in psychotherapy describe their perceptions and experiences of space and time *very* differently. The experience of space and time does not depend upon the measure, the physical, tangible aspect, or the objective limit of it. What does it depend on?

When we are at play, space and time are themselves affected, experientially, by the quality of play, as we said. If play is fun, then time and space tend to feel good, open, free. Time passes quickly. If play turns frustrating, demanding, stressful, intense, then space and time become like a prison sentence, with no release date. The atmosphere turns heavy. The space closes in. Time does not fly.

When fully absorbed in an activity, there is energy and focus, that comes together in what the Hungarian-American psychologist Mihaly Csikszentmihalyi (1990) has called *a flow state*. In this state of being "in the zone" there is a corresponding transformation in your sense of time, almost as if it doesn't exist. There is no need to be aware of space or time as elements of experience.

The value of play, transitional experience, and symbolisation, lies in the opportunity to redress that very quality of lived-experience, if it is at issue. This is also why it is important to open up the Winnicottian notion of play and to extend the application of the idea of transitional phenomena to adults.

Some of Winnicott's case material suggests that he finds a capacity for play in his client's ability to free associate. Is free association a "doing"? I think it is a specialised form of action. It involves an "allowing" if we follow Freud's original instruction (paraphrased as)—*allow to fall freely into your mind whatever happens to, whatever is there for you—allow yourself to put words to this and say whatever lands there without reflection, without selecting or editing out and without censorship. Try not to worry what I might think of it, or how I might judge you. There is a value in our examination of what emerges before we perform any further mental operation upon it.* Here Freud is opening a phenomenological space, prior to reflection, to see what comes up, what appears. It is the right starting point, in my opinion. Then, how will we, mental health professionals, proceed from there?

Playful symbolisation, in Winnicott's sense, is more of an opening up or allowing the possibility of a pre-reflective mind—like a kind of meditation. It occurs in a space and time that is quantifiable, but the experiential quality matters more. Bringing this quality to ordinary living and working releases you from some of the intensity and pressure of your adult responsibilities, needs, and duties. It is not an excuse to be irresponsible. Here you can afford to let your life happen in a way that is enjoyable and rewarding—maybe even easy in relative terms. Without being aware it is happening, the heavy feeling that you must make something happen, achieve something, *be* something, can creep in quietly (at first). You think you are in control, and then you notice you have less and less control in how things unfold. If you get the balance right between what can be controlled and what cannot, and between productivity and doing things for their own sake, it helps to keep your mood uplifted and life on the rails. The aim is to enhance the quality of your experience of living. What is the point of living long if your way of living in not done well or feel agreeable?

I am not advocating a kind of passive or docile attitude. Rather, a way of living becomes possible where you can be receptive to what is there for you. Things don't *have to be* a certain way of your own egocentric or wilful determinations. To some degree, you can be the architect of the design of your life. You have choices. To a large degree, you cannot. If you can accept the limits of what is in your control, you can maintain a personal sense of agency that is effective and autonomous. There is freedom in letting go of how (you thought) it must be; surrender. You are bound to feel mentally healthier.

The implication is not to live without any plan at all but also not to have to adhere rigidly to a plan that is so fully determined that any deviation becomes a crisis. The pandemic has been a lesson in this. Your life is a work in progress. "Life is what happens while you're busy making other plans" (John Lennon). You are neither the architect nor the plan—you reside in between, the potential space for play and symbolisation from which creativity and self-discovery emerge.

* * *

This discussion does not set out to trivialise the terrible suffering of mental illness, nor replace the need for effective treatments, medications, and/or hospital care or other, more intensive interventions. These can be essential, and, accordingly, I refer patients when necessary. Where time for therapy exists, issues of the existential vacuum, meaning, and what makes life worth living can be focused on and the process can mitigate mental suffering, through play and the corresponding experience of embodied symbolisation. I make this disclaimer to ensure the place of mental suffering remains paramount—always. In the context of a truly developmental therapeutic professional relationship, where that is possible and evolving, and through which play and embodied symbolisation occur, the therapy process brings relief and personal growth.

In the example of Judy, the clinical psychologist, and Sean, her eleven-year-old patient, above, their exchanges were charged with energy once they embarked on a word game together and out of that, a meaningful discussion germinated. The conditions for meaning to emerge changed through play leading to symbolisation. Symbolisation *is* a word game. The professional relationship is the occasion and arena for such games to be played in the service of the therapeutic.

Developmental psychotherapy combines the therapeutic treatment of mental suffering with a programme for personal growth, healing from past emotional injury and trauma, and an overcoming of the limitations of earlier development. Will patients choose to join us on a path for growth? And will we, mental health professionals, be up to the challenge?

Part IV

Luke: finding meaning through developmental psychotherapy

CHAPTER 13

Working with Luke: a full-length case study[84]

*To live is to find out for yourself
what is true, and you can do this
only when there is freedom, when
there is continuous revolution
inwardly, within yourself.*
Jiddu Krishnamurti

Introduction

My aim is to bring the ideas of the previous chapters together with a real person, and how we worked together in developmental psychotherapy. There will be some repetition and an echoing of former themes, but here they reside in a clinical context. There are theoretical fragments in the mix that show how ideas of early childhood development apply to adult psychotherapy and the territory of symbol-formation, the origins of attachment, and symbolisation of meaning.

This case has been immensely challenging and raises more questions than I can answer. I have deliberately chosen a difficult case. It is rarely a simple or straightforward business to somehow enable the development of a capacity for meaning-making where formerly there was little, if any at all. Luke deserves credit for persevering when things looked bleak, when there was no reason to have faith in the process. For a long time, I could see no sign of our work

---

[84] With much gratitude to Luke for reading through and allowing me to use this material with few changes or omissions. I have de-identified Luke to protect his privacy.

succeeding or of any reason to believe that something of value would result from years of his battle to find meaning and to feel well.

This long case consists of three sections. Section A is based on the first three and a half years of therapy with Luke (his chosen pseudonym), a single, thirty-seven-year-old Australian man in 2002 when we began. Section B is the culmination of six and a half years total but focusing on a few key moments of the final year, 2009. There were about fourteen intermittent phone sessions over 2010 and until June of 2011. After finishing up, and a gap of almost no contact for four years, Luke returned to therapy in 2015. Our only contact over that time was a few brief emails along the lines of:

> *How are you?*
> *Fine.*
> And once:
> *I should come in and see you.*
> *Yes, please do, it would be good to catch-up when the time is right for you.*
> He didn't.

Section C is about the re-commencement of therapy after a four-year gap from 2015 onwards. Luke's sessions were regular but less frequent than before during this period.

Luke was forty-four years old at the time (2009–2010) I first wrote-up this account, seven years after we first met. We had been working together regularly for twice weekly sessions.

Section A

First impressions (2002)

I remember my very first thought as I saw Luke in my waiting room. Sitting there with a rather severe-looking shaved head, leather jacket, motorcycle helmet on the floor, and wearing an intense frown, he looked rough. I thought *This guy is a serial killer* as I smiled warmly, extended my hand, and introduced myself.

In the first session, Luke said he was seeking therapy because he needed *to untangle his mental state and sort out his relation to his brother.* His brother had been emotionally unstable and mentally ill since his adolescence and had formerly had *massive suicidal depression.* Luke said of himself that he carried too much guilt, he *shovels it onto his plate like an all-day buffet. Guilt about what?* I asked. *Everything and nothing,* he answered.

Luke told me he compulsively looks to meet the needs of others at the expense of himself. He had little energy, no real motivation or authentic sense of what he wanted for himself. He felt miserable most of the time, had low self-esteem, was always feeling apologetic. In his mind, he was always sorry, always saying sorry and often saying sorry out loud. Luke would say the same words over and over again out loud, as if begging forgiveness for something, though it was never quite clear for what. *SORRY BABY LOVE BAD, SORRY BABY KILL LOVE,*

SORRY BABY KILL ME. Disturbing, confusing, enigmatic. Who is speaking to whom? And about what? Why? These questions were never fully answered but hung over Luke's head like a guillotine blade.

He was convinced he always let other people down and was afraid that anyone who got involved with him would get hurt, albeit inadvertently.

Luke told me he was impotent, though he rarely had the opportunity to find out if that had changed. And he felt that he was not growing as a person. I was struck by Luke's way of speaking in a fast monotone, without any variation in pitch, timbre, volume, or pace. The prosody of his voice was always flat.

Otherwise, Luke seemed harmless, if not timid, in contrast to the impression given by his appearance, reinforced over the years. I laughed at myself. Some serial killer! Another example of my amazing intuitive powers.

Many questions arise: is impotence a physical condition or a psychological condition? In my clinical experience, there is usually no discernible underlying organic cause. Is it a symptom or sign of a mental disorder? Is a flat tone of voice such a symptom? Is feeling guilty all the time about everything and nothing? What about saying phrases like *sorry baby* out loud while alone? How should we regard these—as signs of a mental disorder or rather quirky aspects of Luke's personality?

It doesn't help Luke if we tell him he's got a mental disorder. Then what? Medication does not typically make anyone feel less guilty. Not yet.

Theoretical statement

Remembering Winnicott's paradox, I questioned how to approach this work with Luke with "meaning" as a primary reference point. Do we create meaning, or is it there to be found? Does psychotherapy offer meaning like a feed to a hungry baby, or does it have to be discovered or created by the patient? If it is a negotiated process as part of a professional relationship, then how can intersubjective exchange be initiated? For our clinical work, what is happening when there is no meaning to be found or created anywhere? What can anyone do about its absence—the source of so much suffering—as is so often found in the most despairing, withdrawn, and isolated patients?

When patients are damaged, dissociated, suicidally depressed, or entrenched in the existential vacuum, it becomes difficult to adopt an analytic attitude of searching for meaning. Treatment is needed, and very disturbed patients need to be helped to feel better as quickly and directly as possible. In my experience, however, despite their claims and slogans, there are no short-term approaches that make a long-term difference.

It is also not just the longevity of therapy that matters. To develop a capacity for meaningful living, the relationship is the treatment. It is not any relationship. It is not just being *mates*. It is not just the usual qualities of a good counsellor—reflective listening, empathy, understanding, and care—though these are essential. The kind of relationship that makes a difference over time must become a vehicle for transitional experiencing along a journey towards symbolisation, helping patients in coming to terms with their history, present self, life, and way of living.

The middle ground, between yourself and whatever you value or holds meaning, is the area of transitional experiencing. It is neither wholly "inside" nor "outside". If it isn't there at the outset, then you need to remove any obstacles and cultivate a meaningful relationship to create a middle ground. Developmentally, there is a direct continuity from the play area of the child, where child or adult can wrestle with—or play with—possibilities for the endowment of value, of connection, attachment, and meaning. A successful intellectual analysis of these questions is more likely to produce a defensive organisation like that of the false self, or more generally, a kind of living in your head, which already applied to Luke. Living in your head is a formula for isolation. Isolation typically breeds paranoia, loneliness, despair, emptiness, purposelessness—the elements of the existential vacuum, as we said before, and as has been so prevalent in the course of the pandemic.

A transitional object refers to the initiation of the capacity for symbolic experience. Its main function is the creation of a space where value, meaning, interest, and energy can crystallise into being and be felt and held onto—as necessary prerequisites for relatedness. From there, possibilities for intimacy and autonomy open up.

Reiterating: the relationship with the transitional object symbolises what is "me", what is "not me", the connection between, and the differentiation between these two, at once, while none of these should be understood as determinate positions, neither completely fixed nor absolute. One of the difficulties in thinking about these matters is that to have a relationship with an object, that object needs to be psychologically separate from yourself, but separateness is, itself, a major developmental achievement, and judging from the pervasiveness of narcissism, hysterical control, obsessional ordering of the world, and schizoid disorders, it is one that many people never achieve. Add post-traumatic and dissociative disorders, separateness is an elusive wish and mindfulness unachievable. This is the issue to be processed: how can we achieve separateness without disconnectedness? A separateness that remains open and connected allows feeling okay on your own while "meeting" is possible.

In one way of putting it, the transition is from living in a world that is populated by objects and people that are essentially projections of yourself and are conceived-of according to your own design, to a world where otherness and the differences of things and people from yourself can be perceived according to their design. So, it is a transition from conception to perception and a transition from the purely subjective towards objectivity, or put differently, it is also a transition from narcissism to intersubjectivity. A person's potential becomes realisable—made real—as far as possible, as you move through thought and intention to action. In effect, there is a movement out of individual isolation towards being part of a community.

Acceptance, respect, and tolerance for the question of how meaning happens—is it found or created?—leads us to base therapy not on an intellectual analysis but on co-creating ways of promoting a developmental movement where it has stalled.

Case continued—Lost in oblivion (2003)

Returning to Luke, after ten years, he quit his job working for an international company where he was valued for his skills in a highly specialised area of information technology. Since quitting, he had done nothing. He rarely cleaned his house, often didn't eat, open his post, pay bills, or go out. He preferred this to full-time work.

He used to play solo games on the net, just by himself. One of his favourites was called "Oblivion"—an apt metaphor. Yet, while absorbed in Oblivion, Luke undertook many creative tasks, such as writing a complete plot as part of the game. He joined various guilds that involved meaningful work, building environments and communities. There was even a thieves' guild for creative ways of stealing and getting away with it. I am still inclined to see all this as an example of object relating because of its virtual reality. I think object use could involve the same activities but in the lived world. Doing it. (I suppose we will have to confront this distinction increasingly with the advent of the metaverse—virtual worlds that replicate lived experience but in an online realm).

For a while, Luke played a game that involved a whole group of other people, and he became a team leader, which he regarded as a developmental achievement. They spoke together virtually and planned tactics and manoeuvres. They arranged times to meet online for campaigns and, at one stage, the local group met in the flesh for a literal beer in the actual pub. That is object use.

I saw Luke primarily as displaying a schizoid personality structure. He lived largely in fantasy and claimed to feel practically no emotion ever. I have rarely had a patient who could remember so little of his childhood, nothing before fourteen years of age. His description of growing up was: there were four blobs, my mother, father, and an older brother and sister, and that was it.

Before Luke was conceived, his mother consulted a clairvoyant and was told that her third child would be a genius. She admitted to harbouring fantasies that this would lead to a glamorous destiny for her in America. When Luke was born, she knew he was a genius and treated him accordingly. By the time he had finished high school, Luke had largely fulfilled the prophesy and was top of the school, coming first in all seven subjects. He said he was a total nerd who wore thick glasses and a heavy overcoat with the hood pulled up over his head (like *Mr Robot* (2015) before the series screened), more of a character than a person.

I grew to see Luke's addiction to internet gaming as something like a transitional phenomenon. It was something that he used to relieve anxiety and guilt and sometimes even spent a few hours at it if he wasn't tired enough for sleep. Interestingly, one game involved constructing himself into an online character. He incorporated fantasy aspects of himself like the superhero, saving, healing, and rescuing everyone.

Luke could find himself at a complete loss as to how to use a session or what to talk to me about. I harboured a fear that without improvement he might descend into a schizophreniform illness of psychotic proportions or alternatively, deteriorate in the more depressive direction of his elder brother who had been psychotic in the past.

In therapy, there was a long period of time when I frequently felt at risk of passing out, way beyond my normal tiredness. I felt as if I was being psychically drawn into a dead space. I never did pass out, but I had to fight hard to stay awake and alive. After a long period of feeling like that, I realised I had to do something about it. In that state, I was unable to reflect upon what was happening. To overcome this, I made a concentrated effort to focus my mind, and crystal-lise my own psychical resources to reflect upon what I was feeling (or the lack of it) and what it meant. This was more natural to my mental functioning but required unusual effort.

I realised the dead-tiredness stopped me from feeling motivated to undertake therapeutic work, as though it was easier just to coast along with him than to reflect, to formulate thoughts or feelings, to raise them for our mutual exploration and interpretation. This, in turn, gave us the veneer of a relationship without the experience of exchange. Of course, preferring not to work was also exactly what Luke was doing in his own life. That was fair enough for him, but I was there to work. I had to awaken the part of myself that held this motivation and desire and, at the same time, address the transference and countertransference[85] between us, explicitly. The more I did this, the more energised and awake I felt, and the more the therapy became enlivened.

As far as we have been able to surmise, Luke's mother was probably emotionally dead to him for much of his early childhood and subsequent life.[86] He had the impossible task of trying to work out how to relate to a dead object and how to receive emotional nutriment (reminiscent of Tronick's "still face" study). How do you separate out what is "me" from "not me" in those conditions! The transference/countertransference constellation of dynamics in our relation-ship frequently revolved around these themes and the corresponding difficulty of establishing an intersubjective process where a genuine experience of exchange was possible in a fresh and alive present tense. Partly, my job was to revive myself and stay alive.

Through my direct experience of this sort of emotional deadness, I also discovered some-thing of the effects of dissociation in Luke and then in myself, specifically, of how dissociation destroys the capacity for reflection and drains energy, desire, and motivation.[87]

The more Luke included me and let me into his world, the more our relationship involved transitional experiencing. I certainly felt better. I'm not sure if *he* did, but I think he felt some difference, too. Sometimes therapists must cure themselves of the effects that patients have on them in order for the therapy to work.

---

[85] Transference and countertransference are technical terms in psychoanalysis. This is a huge subject but for the sake of brevity, both terms refer to a recurrence of the past in the present. Countertransference refers to the ways that therapists are affected by their patients.

[86] Christopher Bollas suggested this perspective in a private conversation about an earlier iteration of this case study. He was probably thinking of André Green's classic psychoanalytic theory of "the dead mother" complex that describes Luke's psychology quite accurately. The dead mother is not literally deceased but refers to a mother whose emotional engagement has been withdrawn, creating a depression in the child in its wake. (See Green, 1986, Chapter 7—"The Dead Mother", pp. 142–173.)

[87] For more on this, see Bromberg (1998).

When I did find my way into Luke's virtual world, I realised that the game he most played was a war game. Luke was on level 100 out of 100. And his character was one of the most efficient killers of enemy soldiers, monsters, and bosses, as they're called, of all players, globally. "Ah", I blurted out, "you are a serial killer, I knew it", though doubting the wisdom of this outburst. Luke said he loved killing; it was the one thing he can do without feeling guilty about it. He is so afraid of hurting people in real life that it was incredibly enjoyable to decimate other characters in the game, then decimate them again once re-born, and not have to worry about it. Indeed, the other members of his team greatly valued his skills. Noticing a difference in prosody now, when speaking about the campaigns to capture treasures and slaughter bosses, because Luke's tone of voice had a sense of climax, I said "Perhaps this is where you are putting your potency, in a place where you can consummate your own desire, have an impact on another, without having to feel guilty or worry." Usually, Luke didn't appear affected by what I said to him, but this time he looked a bit stunned. He paused, then looked up, smiled broadly, and said "You could sell snake-oil!"

It was dawning on me that the split in Luke between, on the one hand, being harmless, concerned about how men treated women, anguished about how women had suffered because of such mistreatment, and also dismayed by how the environment was being destroyed by so-called civilised men, and, on the other, his love of virtual killing, his exceptional skill at it, and the way this relieved anxiety and guilt, meant something crucial for our work.

Luke could not tolerate his own destructive feelings and impulses and did everything he could to rid them from his system or to bury them so deeply, they *felt* gone. Could his unintegrated destructiveness and hate be an underlying source of his intense, persistent guilt feelings? Guilt over disavowed intentions, rather than acts? Guilt over past feelings now divorced from the present? And so massively *sorry*?

His immersion in online gaming created a potential space in which he could form relationships with other people without worrying that his destructive impulses would be harmful; indeed, they were a valued asset in the context of the war game.

Theory continued—Creating potential space

I was anxious to cultivate a potential space between us through our work in therapy. Potential space is complicated, it is a separation that is also not a separation. It refers to the play of separateness and connectedness that we feel in the interplay between emotional dependency and autonomy. This applies to babies and their carers, adults and each other, and patients and their therapists.

Remember the earlier example of how, when mother leaves the room, a potential space opens up for the baby through the mother's presence and then absence. In this example, if baby becomes anxious and cannot continue playing, there is no potential space. When baby can continue playing without undue anxiety and gets interested in something in the room, potential space exists. There is no need for baby to get preoccupied in mental activity.

In a different example, an adult woman felt more secure when her husband was in bed with her. When he was away, he would phone to say *good night*. When they hung up, she felt more aware of his absence than his presence. The loss of this connection is a loss of potential space. "He" had become a fleeting idea as soon as she was disconnected from his actual voice. Potential space would refer to the feeling of the connection remaining after the phone call has ended.

In a sense, the baby that can make use of potential space continues to feel connected, to feel a sense of mother's presence despite her absence. So, there is a separation that is not a separation because this baby can be separate and autonomous for a time. Here separateness means connection. This can pertain equally to adults as for the woman who felt disconnected when she finished on the phone with her husband. The connection was lost, in both senses.

How is this capacity for lasting connection developed? Again, we know both from parenting and from successful psychotherapy, that there is an experience of trust and reliability, of safety and care, and of attention and love that breeds confidence that can be internalised as a secure sense of self with a relatively peaceful mind and relaxed body. Echoing Chapter 10, this is a good basis for secure attachment, itself the ground of potential space. Contrastingly, when dependency fails, there is a loss in the child's interest in play, the absorption in the child's activity wanes, and there is a corresponding loss of the meaningful symbol.

> Transitional experiencing initiates engagement
> with a meaningful symbol.

What does "meaningful symbol" mean? It refers to any object, activity, or relationship that holds value or meaning for you. The lack or loss of it leads to emptiness, whereas abundance of meaningful symbols gives a feeling of fullness.

Although Luke is not in a crisis, his whole life seems like something of a crisis of meaning and purpose. Luke's childhood does not appear to contain any trauma that he can remember but some people's whole childhood is traumatic. Could growing up with an emotionally dead mother be such a trauma? Could simply not being seen for who you are, right from the start, also be a trauma? And one that forecloses the possibility of potential space, as a consequence? A lack of felt-connection can be a traumatising deprivation even if all material needs are well met. *You don't know what you're missing.*

For the adult, we can see how potential space is operating, or how it isn't, through cultural experiences. It doesn't matter if you get lost in listening to Mozart or Metallica, or if you live for the football or Shakespeare, or love to spend your time gardening, writing poetry, or trading digital assets. And there is a potential space in the consulting room. What will a patient make of it? Is there something this patient can get into with me, and without me having to do something or instruct, direct, or guide them into what I think is important? When there is no potential space between us, nothing of interest or redeemable in the world to be discovered, nothing or no one to play with, that is a condition in need of treatment. Sadly, this has largely been the case with Luke. The online war game is the exception.

Luke became interested in his own dreams and discovered I was interested, too. We began to play with his dreams in therapy. In this sense, play and work and transitional experiencing became synonymous. A potential space was opening up through our discussions of his dreams. Then, he recorded something of our discussions in his journal, even if he calls it snake oil. We seemed to mirror each other in taking copious notes—something felt important, compelling, maybe even meaningful.

Case continued—Integrating hate (2004)

In one session Luke reported the following dream after another period of weeks during which the therapy felt noticeably flat or lifeless:

> A fat, self-important turd of a police officer insisted upon giving me a fine of $150 for walking out on a red, do-not-walk signal. I hate his guts. He has insisted on my filling out details for him. He's making me do the work of incriminating myself. As I pull out my wallet to pay the fine, bits of paper fall out and the police officer threatens to get me on a littering charge as well. As I fill out the form, I accidentally put my foot on it, and it rips down the middle. I have a stab of anxiety about that as well.
>
> The next image has no apparent connection with the first part. I have a large plastic tube of water with an ogre's finger joint in it with a pointed fingernail like a claw. The finger is suspended in there like a cork floating in water.

I asked Luke for any associations to the dream. It occurred to him that maybe the water in the tube represented emotion, specifically the tears that he had not cried despite being in therapy for a number of years at this point. Yes, I could see that.

While I wasn't in a big hurry to associate myself with the image of a fat, self-important turd of a police officer I said that nevertheless $150 was the fee that he was paying me. I do take notes and make him do work and he often feels incriminated. I wondered if he felt like he littered his sessions with bits and pieces of himself and sometimes feels like he puts his foot in it. Sometimes, his form as a person seems torn. In the dream, he said he hates the police officer's guts, but I don't see much expression of hating my guts apart from occasional indirect or joking insults like the snake-oil comment.[88]

This interpretation led to a full and frank discussion in which Luke could say that he had felt extremely frustrated with the therapy, with the feeling of it dragging and how little change or

---

[88] This is an example of a transference interpretation.

progress he felt from it. I said perhaps this is also a measure of how long it is taking to trust me enough to bring more of his feelings into it even if that makes him feel vulnerable.

Therapy has had a different feel since then, not completely different, but certainly less flat or dead. It felt important that I could receive his "hate" and rather insulting representation in the dream without feeling hurt or humiliated or retaliatory and correspondingly, for him not to have to feel guilty or sorry about it. This is an example of "destroying the object" and the importance of the object (me) surviving, not retaliating, and not being destroyed completely.

Thinking about dissociation—there is usually an intensely hostile internal environment where patients attack, criticise, and typically put themselves down (remember Clarissa from Chapters 3 and 5). It is as if the dissociated person needs to punish themselves for being dissociated, because dissociation itself makes it so hard to feel well and to feel that it is okay "to be me exactly as I am". As I see it, Luke's fear of the inevitability of hurting anyone has to do with his inclination to project this punishing, insulting, and attacking part of himself. He fears hurting someone and fears their retaliation. So, a dream like the one above is important in bringing this to light.

Theory continued—A phenomenology of dissociation

I see many patients who do not recall having experienced trauma[89] in any discrete sense and yet in whom dissociation is rife. Emotional neglect and abuse are insidious. Luke is one example.

In therapy, dissociation shows itself through enactment while manifesting as an omission from patients' narratives. Luke's insults to me are both a projection and an enactment. My difficulty in keeping my attention focused upon his discourse is also an example of a countertransference enactment, as was my dead-tired feeling of nearly passing out.

Previously, therapists were trying to help people to remember. Now, we understand that what has been dissociated cannot be remembered but rather needs to be re-membered, a putting together of what remains unsymbolised. The space between dissociated parts of yourself takes on an existence when the space becomes a potential space, and its absence has a presence. Transitional experiencing bridges the gaps between dissociated states and spaces.

The difficult question, at least for me, is how can we enable the symbolisation of that which has never been symbolised? It has never been symbolised either because the experience of emotional neglect, abuse, injury, or even shock occurred before there was language to express it or because dissociation rendered the person absent to their experience in a way that makes later reflection upon it impossible. There are literally no words if the experience occurred

---

[89] Emotional neglect is possibly the most common and most damaging form of early trauma, though nothing is specifically "done to" the child. If anything, not enough is done—as in direct engagement and care. Dissociation may also occur to prevent a feeling of being unsafe in the early attachment relationship. Its primary function is protection.

prior to the acquisition of language. Dissociation prevents remembering the feelings associated with early trauma in the attachment relationship. It's helpful to consider dissociation phenomenologically.

Something serious has happened but you feel nothing. When asked about it, you give a report of it as if it happened to someone you've never met, like in a newspaper story. If you find yourself in a similar situation again, you become psychically paralysed, and then later wake up and return to normal as if emerging from a trance state, largely unaware of where you've been, what happened, or what it means.

You switch from one state or mood or theme in your thinking to another without being aware that a switch has occurred. It is as if there were a rule: you can go down a particular mental track just so far and then you must jump ship and proceed in another direction. But there is also a meta-rule that says you will not be aware of that first rule. So, the act of jumping ship itself is not recognised, like a post-hypnotic suggestion. Putting it differently, dissociation, like a computer virus, has built into it a means of avoiding detection. It is the negation of the part of yourself that enables you to register this very negation. The ontological status of dissociation is non-existence, giving another dimension to the meaning of the unconscious. It is not simply a non-existence; rather, it is something that *should* exist and have a place in your conscious experience. It is a hole in the fabric of experiencing, a vortex—an existential vacuum. Something is missing and so cannot be conceived of. Inconceivable means unthinkable.

> Because dissociation is unthinkable,
> it is also unspeakable.

The clinical implications of transitional experiencing indicate a need to facilitate the transition from the unsymbolised and unsymbolisable to something that can be thought, felt, reflected upon, and spoken of. The act of jumping ship needs to become able to be recognised via reflection. This enables a transition from dissociation to intra-psychic conflict, and from a hidden reality that exists in one person but affects others to an issue that can be owned as part of a relationship. So, this is also a transition from subjectivity, once you are formed enough to be a subject, to intersubjectivity, from an individual self to relationship, and from intra-being to inter-being.

Here is how Bromberg puts it:

> It is the "room for relatedness" that turns static, frozen space into "potential space", and allows the creative encounter between a patient's multiple realities and those of his analyst to form into something new—a negotiated enhancement of the patient's perceptual

capacity and an increased surrender of the dissociative structure of his personality organisation. (1998, p. 217)

Transitional experiencing is an idea that refers to a professional relationship that cultivates the conditions necessary for personal development. It is not a point about clinical technique. I say things to patients that they do not hear, indeed cannot hear. I try to show them things that they cannot see. And I try to reach them and touch them somewhere deep in themselves, but they cannot feel it. It is also clear to me that this happens in reverse with respect to my own deaf, blind, and numb areas. It works both ways; if you cut me off, then I am cut-off, and vice versa.

First, you have to overcome being cut-off from the cut-off if you are ever to produce a good-enough therapeutic relationship where transitional experiencing does its work and dissociation, and isolation are overcome as far as possible in the service of emotional engagement and developmental growth. Failing to notice that you've failed to notice is another way of saying: cut-off from being cut-off.

The aim of dissociation is to disrupt the continuity of experience so that you are never caught off guard again for the possibility of attack from without. One of the key paradoxes of dissociation is that its aim is to create safety by making it impossible to ever relax. By remaining mentally hypervigilant and emotionally hyperaroused, you protect a dead space and can never feel safe. The purpose of dissociation is protection, but what you protect yourself from (living freely, openly, unguarded) is what you *actually* need to feel safe.

> Dissociation destroys the possibility of the illusion
> of safety in the act of trying to create it.

Michael Eigen, one of the early relational theorists, puts it like this in his paper called "The area of faith in Winnicott, Lacan and Bion":

> The subject here, as in transitional experiencing, grows through paradoxical rather than dissociative awareness. (1999, p. 10)

Paradoxical awareness, and a capacity to hold such contradictions, even without resolution, enables the past to be linked with the present; and to be present, without excessive charge—the Freudian term for this is *decathexis*—reducing the energy in the intense feeling of threat. Too much therapeutic attention is spent on trying to cure our patients of what was done to them in the past that made them feel unsafe, or traumatised, in the first place. Paraphrasing Bromberg:

in understanding why a therapeutic cure is not lasting, we understand that we cannot cure patients of what was done to them in the past; rather, we are trying to cure them of what they still do to themselves and to others in the present, to *cope* with what was done to them in the past and how it still affects them (1992, p. 217).

What I have found when there has been some success in overcoming dissociation is that patients then have to climb a Mount Everest of regret that is built upon the realisation of how much has been missed and wasted. This is depressing, but what is needed is an opportunity for grieving.

Through many subsequent discussions with Luke, it became clear that Luke felt sorry for having sexual feelings and desires, and that he worried greatly that his sexuality could be harmful to others. Like so many dissociated people, he felt a deep sense of shame. It also became clear that the frequent phases of deadness in the therapy occurred as a consequence of his difficulty in bringing both his sexuality and his destructiveness into our sessions for fear they could not be contained, and would be too much to bear.

Case Continued—From self-hate to play (2005)

Luke reported this dream in a session about three and a half years into therapy:

> I am running my finger around the anus of a naked young lady lying on her front. And that's the dream.

"What do you think it means?" I ask.

"I don't know", he replies. [*Pause*] "Maybe it means I'm an asshole."

"Is that all you can think of?" I ask, looking a bit sceptical.

"Well, what do you think?" he challenges me.

I have no thought in my head at all but I hear myself say: "Maybe there can be pleasure felt in making contact with the place where shit happens?"

He smiles broadly and quips: "Nice one, I'm really getting my money's worth today."

"Cheers", I reply, doubting this was a compliment. "C'mon, it's your turn. Can you add anything to that?"

I am trying to invite him to reflect with me through the sort of playful banter that has become more common between us. My patient's first thought of his dream is to put himself down and call himself an asshole in a way that fits the self-effacing pattern I mentioned before. What I am trying to do is to invite him out of his customary, solitary, and hostile internal environment into a different environment with me where we can play with ideas, reflections, and associations meaningfully—where we can associate rather than dissociate, where we can associate together rather than be assholes alone.

Transitional experiencing means building a relationship as a context and a process for new experiences, where it is safe-enough to afford the possibility of connectedness both within oneself and between us as a medium of healing and a pathway of recovery.

> ## Then the past can have a living presence.

Even the worst past can feel benign if you can put it behind you (easy to say, I know, but look at Frankl!). Then, a therapeutic relationship is built with work and play in the present. Therapeutic work gives it substance and play gives it meaning; both make it feel like a purposeful, even enjoyable, activity. That is how the present comes to feel benign. This sounds idealistic, but it is desirable nonetheless.

Eigen says:

> In transitional experiencing primordial symbolisation takes the form of an affective cognition in which self-other awareness creatively thrives. *Self-other awareness is itself the core of symbolising experiencing* and perhaps remains humankind's most creative activity at various levels of developmental complexity. (1999, pp. 15–16, original emphasis)[90]

Eigen is indicating that relationships that enable transitional experiencing require integrating both thinking and feeling in the creative endeavour of separating out what is "me" from what is "not me". Then, giving voice and expression to the meaning of your experience follows.

Case continued—Feeling, together

Later, in this same session, Luke said that over the weekend he was home by himself and feeling miserable as usual when he remembered I had said I could see he had spent much of his life really suffering. His eyes watered when he thought of that at home and, indeed, in the session a single tear welled up, and rolled down his cheek as I watched. That was the first tear in over three and a half years. A single, saline droplet of solitary testimony to his now-felt pain. I felt it, too, and a single tear welled up in my eyes and rolled down my cheek. Without thinking about it, it was as if my emotional/physiological system was synchronised to his and was mirroring back his/my feelings in a mutually expressed pre-symbolic, transitional moment that was itself

---

[90] By "primordial symbolisation takes the form of an affective cognition" I understand Eigen to mean the earliest "transitional" experiences of symbolisation take the form of felt-thought, thinking with feeling or even thinking through feeling in the baby's awareness of others.

a reflection of our reflections.[91] Somehow, the interval between our sessions had been bridged and informed by this feeling of pain—a pain connected to its object—on the way to the affective cognition that Eigen speaks of.

Luke was experiencing something of an emotional nature that was happening in the present. His feeling, his tear, was connected to something I had said that he was remembering. It wasn't the abstract, programmed misery that had been so customary.

At this point, despite the signs of an emotional life beginning to emerge in a more poignant way, Luke was feeling deeply despondent about a girl he was interested in who told him she was interested in someone else. He seemed deeply sad and disappointed and said "I feel like I am in permanent exile". I thought to myself, Luke never begins speaking with *I feel*. Lately, I notice Luke's voice bears no resemblance to the former monotone but rather is varied in volume and tone and full of colour—no less so than in the following exchange.

> Luke said he is in a self-imposed withdrawal from other people.
>
> I said: "It is painful when you want someone, and they don't want you back in the same way."
>
> He said: "I had the thought that I just want to be somewhere else. I should just get out of here."
>
> I said: "Maybe that is a metaphor for wanting to be somewhere other than where you are, in yourself?"
>
> He exclaimed: "Yes, of course! Why do you think I play so many video games? To be somewhere else."
>
> I said: "Perhaps your feelings have also been exiled though you do seem to be feeling more today …"
>
> He said impatiently: "Yes, we know this…"
>
> Luke can make me feel like such an idiot. I said: "Sorry, I feel like I've stated the obvious, again."
>
> Luke replied: "Now you're sorry and I feel sorry that I've made you feel sorry, and I feel like I should say sorry for that."
>
> And I said: "Now I feel sorry that I've made you feel sorry for making me feel sorry and I want to say sorry to you for that …" and we both started laughing at the sheer absurdity of what we had got into.[92]

---

[91] You can put this down to mirror neurons, but the brain science represents such a phenomenon as mechanical whereas the experience felt meaningful, emotionally.

[92] As he read a draft of this chapter, at this juncture Luke said: "You know, you don't have to worry about stating the obvious or bringing up something again—just do it, because it's always helpful and it doesn't matter if we've talked about it before." I found this helpful, too, and good to know—and said so. And though the chapter was finished, this also indicated that our work would go on.

Case continued—A potent space for sexuality: overcoming shame (2006)

After that session, Luke decided to have a birthday party, invited people over, cleaned his house, and went out to buy drinks and snacks and music. He also went and booked a session with a prostitute during which he maintained an erection and seemed to have quite a good time. He said that while he was happy about that, it was also hard for him to enjoy the sex without worrying if it was good for her.

I said:	"You seem to be making a transition from an online community to an actual community and a transition from porn on the net to sex with a real person."
He said:	"The sexual experience had lacked intimacy and emotional attachment. I blurted out You can't expect that from one meeting with a sex worker."
He countered by saying:	"Actually, while in the missionary position, I looked into her eyes and she looked back into mine and I felt we had made contact there, for an instant, as two people."
I said:	"That sounds worth something. Hey, I'm curious. How much did you have to pay for this?"
He said:	"Twice as much as I pay you." And I quipped: "Now I'm really feeling sorry."
He said, accusatorily:	"Yeah, well you didn't let me come in your mouth in the first session."
I said:	"No, you're going to have to wait a long time for that to happen. But I do let you come in my ears …"

My point in talking "dirty" is to say that somehow in the play of sexuality and the intercourse of our speech, both in Luke's life and between us, it is becoming possible for Luke to be a sexual being, without having to feel he is bad or harmful and without having to feel shame, guilt, and remorse. It was important that he could tell me about his sexual experience, indeed achievement, without being judged, or feel undue fear about the possibility of it. I felt more of a sense of connection between us. Accordingly, Luke's life seemed to be starting to feel worth living—to him. He said so.

This is where we had arrived by the end of 2006. Now, I want to jump to 2009, our sixth year. If I leap over 2007 and 2008, it doesn't mean that nothing happened over those years. Luke spent a great deal of time expressing his concern over the state of the world, especially the deterioration of the natural environment and his grave fears for a cataclysmic environmental disaster that is inevitable from his point of view. Luke often seemed to feel single-handedly responsible for the state of the world and responsible for fixing it, though he never actually did anything of a practical nature at this stage.

Section B

Telling dreams: the symbolisation of the core issue (2009)

Luke returned from an overseas trip and was surprised to discover that he could not return to his former job as he had often done in the past. The global financial crisis had struck, and he was out of work, having spent all his savings travelling. For much of the first half of the year, Luke was depressed, anxious, and occasionally had suicidal ideation. Having time on his hands and no money was not a formula for happiness, though Luke did manage to continue therapy.

I wasn't sure if he should continue therapy under those circumstances. Sometimes it is hard even for therapists to believe how important therapy is for their patient, when evidence of benefit is faint, and the cost has grown as people can afford less than before.

Luke came in one day saying that he could barely stay engaged or pay attention to practically anything for more than fifteen minutes at a time.

> I asked: "What engages you most now?"
>
> He answered: "It used to be online war games and porn but neither does it for me now. I'm still avoiding my life!" and went on to describe how the world had seemed quite a hopeful place to him as a child, where good things could happen, and joy was possible. As he got older, he found that the world was seriously fucked, bent on a self-destructive course, that probably nothing can reverse. So, he hides in his cave, waiting for it all to fall apart, feeling guilty for not doing anything about it.
>
> I said: "You must have felt the world that emerged as you grew up was a massive betrayal and disappointment."
>
> Luke nodded, noticeably tearing up. I was feeling a strong current of emotional pain and thinking how devastating this turning from hopeful to hopeless must have been for him. Despite the relative lack of positive emotions, at least Luke was able to feel something of an emotional nature. This is, after all, the converse of dissociation.

By the end of May I was feeling despondent about Luke's therapy. The amount of time did not appear to have helped Luke "enough", his internal battles, his lack of motivation, his perpetual isolation, still sorry, still guilty, and not making good use of his time or our sessions. He spoke about wanting a girlfriend, sex, and company but then would do nothing about it, often not replying to communications from women who had responded to his profile on one of the online dating websites.

It is tempting to spin theory to suit your own way of understanding things, but now I found myself questioning and doubting the value of all these years of work and wondering if there was ever going to be some tangible manifestation of improvement both in Luke's "internal" world and his "external" relations and activities. There had been some small signs of development, but it was getting harder and harder for me to keep faith in the value of the process as he appeared to be going downhill despite the optimistic implications of my ideas about development.

In 2006, I had written a paper on the first three years of his therapy. And in 2009, I wanted to write a follow-up paper on the next three years of therapy but with little to show for it, few tangible improvements, what kind of paper could I write? After six and a half years of therapy with Jan Resnick, his patient wants to kill himself. That's a great paper. And hang the paper, what about the patient?

Then the following session occurred (Session No 434) on 28 May 2009. Luke begins with a dream he had written down and this is a verbatim account of how he told it to me.

> I am in a school or university. Someone needed me to reformat a computer. They needed some data from the computer first. I was supposed to have collected this data.
>
> I was looking through a loose-leaf binder to see if I had the data. Someone gave me some additional information and I said "Wait a minute, this isn't the data. This is the list of what the data should be but not the data itself."
>
> I'm still looking for this data and can't find it. Then I am looking at a high-walled Indian fortress, in Gandhara. It is an unexplored region on an island. What I need is in there. But it is like a section of a video game that I haven't even played, a level I haven't reached yet. I've got to play this game through in order to find this high-walled fortress, in order to get the information I need, that I am supposed to get off this computer before I do the reformatting.
>
> Getting the data is only one task amongst many that I am supposed to be doing. "I'm screwed." [*He tells me this means that there is no way he can see how to get this data from inside the fortress*] I wake up.
>
> The feeling that I have upon awakening is one of CRUSHING RESPONSIBILITY.

Luke informed me that Gandhara is from the 1978 TV series *Monkey*[93] he watched as a kid. Gandhara is a place where the Buddhists kept their scriptures, a destination for the pilgrims who journeyed from the West (the specific implication here is to discover enlightenment). Something from childhood is emerging into consciousness.

> He is hung up on the thought that everything he does when unenlightened is futile, is just a perpetuation of human suffering. Then, he says, he is thinking of Krishnamurti (knowing I am familiar with Krishnamurti's writings) who says that a revolution in the external world is pointless without a revolution of your heart and mind. You will just repeat the mistakes humanity already made before.[94]

---

[93] Originally, a Japanese television drama series called *Saiyūki*, literally *Account of the Journey to the West* and often mistakenly called *Monkey Magic* due to the show's title song.

[94] "Those who haven't learned from history are doomed to repeat it."

I say:	"There seems to be something in yourself that you need to find, in an unexplored region of yourself."
He replies:	"Oh, I see, you are taking this dream as an allegory of my entire self."
I say:	"Yes, there is this task that you must complete in order to fulfil another task, the finding of data before re-formatting the computer. After you wake up—you feel this sense of crushing responsibility, all of this is before you can really start living …"
He says:	"Enlightenment."
I say:	"Yes, as if you have to be enlightened before you can proceed with anything, in order for it to have a value."

At this point, it occurs to Luke to say that he has been thinking about this: "How can we disappoint ourselves? I am the self who is doing the disappointing as well as the self who is disappointed. It's only possible if you are already split against yourself."

He pauses, looks thoughtful, and then quotes a book he had been reading earlier: "It is only from the innermost silences of the heart that we know the world and what the world has made us."

I had been indicating that there was no task that needed to be accomplished, that this is the hang-up, that he has been expecting something impossible of himself before he begins to live, something that had to be done that is not achievable and prevents him from living actively, in a more involved way, through direct emotional engagement with the world.

Luke responded:	"You mean there is no task, the reformatting of my self that I've been seeking is a paradox; it lies in realising no reformatting is needed in order to be myself. There is nothing that has to be done or discovered; I just have to allow all of that to fall away from me, and then the reformatting will have happened, organically, of its own accord?"
I say:	"Yes! Absolutely! The discovery is that there is nothing to discover. The snow goose does not have to bathe its feathers to make them white. Why should you have to make an effort to be yourself?" [*Here, I am excited and repeating back to him a quote from Lao Tzu that he gave to me a few sessions earlier*] I paused and then I went on. "The data is data-less, there is no information you need to be yourself, no walls to scale, no fortress to penetrate, no task." There was a long, silent pause, contemplating this, and then, in a fashion all too familiar to me, Luke said … "Maybe".

After we finished there was a powerful sense that something had happened, like never before. Being able to symbolise the split for himself meant being able to hold both parts at once, to hold the contradiction without having to resolve it, a separation that connects. The conceptualisation of the split and the ability to reflect on both parts of it together suggests that the dissociative tendency is letting go. Dissociation is the negation of the part of yourself that would enable you to register this very negation. That is the difference; there is a registration of a split that is no longer negated. In noticing, he has overturned the failure to notice. There is a relation that connects where formerly there was an opposition that divides. And *we* felt more connected in a different way.

The sense of exchange that had been lacking was emerging in this intersubjective space. Ideally, in psychoanalytic therapy, patients arrive at their own understandings. This is what autonomy means in practice. Often, many patients are not there, especially in the early stages, not ready or able to forge these meaningful connections that shed light on complex issues. This is a maieutic process, to use a Socratic term: intellectual and emotional midwifery, drawing out latent thoughts and feelings, in the service of emotional engagement. From there, the movement of understanding is dialectical, like dancers moving to the music of intersubjective exchange.

My experience of working with dreams has shown that when a dream emerges that feels important, a revelation of something new that needs to be realised, even if it appears in the codified form of the dream-scape (imagery and language), an opportunity is presented to interpret its symbolic meaning. It has emerged at the point in time when the dreamer is ready to embrace the insight and process its deeper meaning. Often, though cryptic, it holds the exact indication needed for change and development to unfold from there.

Later, I was reflecting on the session, and I remembered that I had had an important insight for myself in my own therapy. I had seen that I had been expecting way too much of myself and feeling disappointed at not achieving what I had hoped. I saw that I had projected this on practically everything of importance in my life, including my children, my partner, The Churchill Clinic (the training organisation that I had founded and ran for eighteen years), and even my patients. Then, I considered the timing of these events.

I had that realisation during a therapy session of my own the week before, on Friday, 22 May. Luke told me he had woken with his Gandhara dream on the Saturday morning, 23 May. Could it be that here, our respective intra-psychical processes appear to be linked in a kind of parallel process? We seem to have triggered something in each other that occurred separately but at about the same point in time, in a potential space between us. Or should we see this as an example of Jungian synchronicity?

There is a curious metaphysic to human relationships where we seem to be connected despite spatial or temporal distance. When we are connected, then space and time lose their function of separating, sequencing, and differentiating. There is a transcending of the material limits of space and time, and, in the process, a self-transcendence.[95] Could it be that such metaphysical, inter-psychic, connections are what make space and time become potential space and potential time?

The next week, we discussed the Gandhara dream in Luke's session. Later, that night I went to sleep and woke with a dream of my own, the only dream in which Luke figures.

---

[95] Of which Frankl speaks.

I am going off on a trip in my dream. I am due at the airport at 9 a.m. or 9-something. We have arranged that Luke will drive me there. I am anxious to be there in good time.

There was a sense that I was going off to a glamorous event, perhaps to give a speech, and that I was rather well-known.

This dream followed the day's session with him which felt like a breakthrough to me. Something of his former dissociation had let go, and his split-self came together to some degree. *Maybe*.

In my dream, I was using Luke to get me somewhere. I had been thinking about presenting a paper at a psychiatry conference on the other side of the country based on my work with Luke. His mum also came to mind. The theme of taking flight felt to me like an expression of my desire to get away from my own despondency about this case, perhaps as Luke's mum had felt during his childhood, both of us seeking an alternative, idealised world rather than immersion in what was actually happening. Perhaps both of us saw Luke as a vehicle to transport us to a better life?

Etymologically, the word "happening" shares the same Old Norse root *happ*—meaning *chance, fate,* or *good luck*—as the word "happy". In one way of looking at it, happiness requires us to be congruent with what is happening. For Luke, I was anxious that he move from a hapless and hopeless place, and for myself, I was not happy this hadn't happened. (Our egocentric desire and impatience for patients to get "better" obstructs their simply being—and their ability to dwell in that "place" long enough for the movement of development to happen.)

Case continued—Breakdown and breakthrough: towards embodiment (2009)

Then, a surprising session occurred (9 June). Luke told me he'd been re-reading a children's book from his childhood called *We Didn't Mean to go to Sea* (Ransome, 1930), and as he was telling me, he became tearful. I asked him to tell me the story in detail. While doing so, Luke broke down more than he ever has with me, or possibly ever.

It is a hopeful story of how children accidently drift out to sea on an otherwise unmanned sailing yacht that loses its mooring. Heroically, they save the boat and, in the process, save themselves before being reunited with their father. Luke is deeply moved through the re-telling of the story to me, with tears streaming down his face. Luke experienced a high level of resonance to his own mental state. As we spoke about hope, Luke indicated that he felt hopeful about a job in Singapore that he had applied for. He also felt hopeful about a couple of women who had responded to his profile on the dating website.

I have the idea that when things change "inside", the "outside" world responds.[96] It might not happen immediately. Often events reflect personal changes and development. Sometimes, things work that didn't work before.

In the very next session (22 June), I heard Luke had been offered the job in Singapore and later, he was offered his old job back, which meant he could stay here. Luke decided to take the

---

[96] It's difficult not to resort to dualistic language, it is so embedded in colloquial use.

job in Singapore; he viewed it as a fresh start and said he hoped "the move would clear out his emotional tubes", as he put it. He thanked me for "getting him here".

Shortly before leaving (7 July), Luke told me that he had smoked some pot and that had given him a liberated feeling and an openness to emotional experiencing unfamiliar to him. He said that he could feel the muscles in his back and feel his spine. Then, suddenly, a surge of feeling welled up from his legs right up through his body. He felt wobbly and bashed his head into the door frame, fell on the floor and cracked up laughing. He noticed that he felt particularly clearheaded as he lay on the floor and felt his entire body reverberating. Then he felt blood and energy surging up his back and into his head. He felt freer in his body than he'd ever felt before; something was moving, something had been released. He felt playful and free, as never before. He felt embodied.

He went out and lay down on the balcony and gazed at the moon and the stars. He said that he felt like he was having a bodily experience of relief. And then looking at me, Luke asks: "Any comment?"

I didn't know what to say but I replied "Well, perhaps you had some kind of epiphany or catharsis—or maybe you were just happily stoned. It's probably the kind of thing that's better assessed down the track looking back at it, but it's still great to hear you feeling a sense of relief, whatever it means, and that you feel more centred in your own body.

He had been to his role-playing group for the last time before moving and told me his character beat someone up and then shat on the other character's head, as his parting shot.

He enjoyed that, but then noticed guilt creeping in. Then he remembered how when he was travelling, he discovered that he could turn his feeling of guilt imaginatively into a large dog that was outside of himself and take the dog for a walk. When he did this, he always felt better.

In one email, a month later in August, Luke wrote that he had been out with a girl a couple of times and had quite a good time. He'd gotten a flat in a lush green area of Singapore and one of the first things he'd done was "collected litter out of the pools in the stream in the nature reserve below my street and shifted rocks that were blocking the flow. It was fulfilling."

A small thing perhaps, but to me, Luke was interacting with the environment to improve it. He has always been so intensely concerned about the environment in the abstract (object relating). Now, at last, there was practical involvement. He was doing something (object use). And it felt fulfilling. Funny how we can feel a sense of fullness from something small.

Interim summary

Summarising the main points:

- This treatment—called developmental psychotherapy—is a relationship and one that can be used by the patient along parallel lines to that of a small child with a transitional object.
- The middle ground between ourselves and the world is the area of transitional experiencing, where meaning and investment of ourselves into "things" that matter can crystallise into

being. The paradoxical nature of meaning—is it inherent or have I put it there?—should be neither challenged nor resolved.

- Therapists need internal radar for dissociation as it often shows itself through both transference and countertransference enactment. This means that it gets acted-upon or acted-out rather than experienced inwardly as something that can be felt, thought about, reflected upon, and raised as a subject for discussion. Dissociation prevents the felt-experience that is the underpinning of aliveness and affective immediacy; qualities that inform mental health and well-being.

- Transitional experiencing is a vehicle for the transformation of what is dissociated and hence unsymbolisable, into intra-psychic conflict (that can be thought) and then be brought into intersubjective exchanges and reflections in the service of making-meaning—and feeling it, feeling that it matters, and speaking, expressing how you feel, in the sense of embodied symbolisation. Thus, embodied symbolisation is a basis for mental/emotional health even if what is felt is painful.

- The developmental pathway towards autonomy and the possibilities for intimacy depend upon building a capacity for symbolisation. Symbolisation is a coming to terms in both senses, coming to terms with things in the sense of acceptance and coming to language, to say what you mean and mean what you say. This is not just a cognitive function but the marriage of cognitive and affective that, itself, signifies development and a recovery, often from trauma, in one sense or other.

Sense + Feeling = Meaning

- Play and, if anything, the emergence of an inner freedom to play, is generative of such capacities for symbolisation and creativity. This has everything to do with feeling well and feeling real. The pot-smoking for Luke was an occasion of play. He turned bumping his head into something playful and funny instead of an occasion for self-pity or misery.

- Through play, symbolising, and transitional experiencing, you move from object relating to object use, interacting with the world rather than fantasising about it or imagining it. Empty, dead space, being at a loose end, not knowing what to do with yourself, not being able to get into anything purposeful, is transformed through the cultivation of a potential space. To make this possible, dissociated, post-traumatic spaces need to be bridged. This can entail opening the floodgates of emotional pain, shame, and depression and then grieving for lost time. Once opened, these painful feelings can be worked through, over time, with sensitivity and compassion. The more worked-through, the greater uplift in mood and available energy, as possibilities for meaningful living open up.

That said, not everyone can open floodgates of emotional pain; for some the pain is too great—but recovery from trauma is still possible. I cannot say the patient with the spider phobia from Chapter 10 *recovered* from his horrendous history of trauma, but he was able to continue therapy with his psychiatrist. I understand the work made more of a difference once they had a better understanding of what they were dealing with. Other patients have recovered well even from extreme histories of complex trauma.

- Potential space is a metaphor for the condition of the possibility of intersubjective exchange, a more connected sense of relationship. This is an avenue with two-way traffic. Therapists must continue to work on themselves as a necessary part of working with others. (This is lacking in mainstream psychology and psychiatry though some recognise the need for their own therapy and undertake it voluntarily. For proper psychoanalytic psychotherapy training, personal therapy is prerequisite; it is part of the foundational ethos of professional practice. Many seasoned therapists return to therapy even late in their careers. Anyone who has not had considerable personal therapy[97] should not call themselves a psychotherapist.)

- In therapy, it is often darkest before the dawn. This requires therapists to hold faith in the value of the process. If you can do that, and hold on to hope for relief, change, and development, then hope becomes possible for your patients to get in touch with. Hope emerges as the emergency recedes.

- Some of the best outcomes of therapy occur after therapy has finished (see Shedler, 2010) or alternatively, are a "sleeper effect" or reflect "negative benefits"—if that doesn't sound like too much of a contradiction. By that, I mean that something adverse that would have happened or used to happen, does not happen, or no longer happens. Luke, though miserable for many years, did not descend into a schizophreniform illness, for example. He could have.

Lastly, as a postscript on the case: I had a phone consultation with Luke in September 2009. He was doing well, going out with a woman, feeling comfortable with that, and he told me he was feeling relatively content. He said he was still muttering under his breath, out loud, when he walked his cool (imaginary) dog named Guilder (meaning "gold"[98]) down the street. Instead of what he had been saying before—"sorry baby love bad"—now he was only saying one word—"love".

By January 2010, Luke still sometimes said "love" out loud but often it was just a sound that began with "luh".

We had fourteen sessions between January 2010 and June 2011. Only one or two were in person, in my consulting room. Most were on the telephone from Singapore. Luke established

---

[97] See, especially, McWilliams (2004, pp. 60–69).

[98] It is significant that Luke turned his depression and feelings of guilt imaginatively into something cool, as he put it, a dog called Guilder or "gold"—he pointed this out to me as he read a draft of this chapter.

a relationship with Jenny, the woman he had been seeing, that raised some new issues while it resolved others. Some key points from those sessions:

- I feel I can be the most varied flavours of myself while role-playing.
- Now I can say "I love you" back to Jenny when she says it to me.
- We are fully sexual; I've had no impotence problems at all.
- I've been happy lately(!)[99]
- Later: sometimes, I have a tension in my body, a scared, panicky feeling in my chest, it's cold, tight, constricted, and colours my experience of the world. Everyone takes on a threatening aspect.
- Later still: while visiting Australia, I got stoned, took off my clothes and lay on my bed, and breathed deeply. I felt my body, got in touch with it and felt it was my own. I felt my heart area and felt all that tightness and constriction around my heart. I associate that with the miserableness when I feel that. I still sometimes wish a meteor would land on my head—it would be a relief.
- He loves being with Jenny—"It's lovely being with her"—I'm happy with her though there are anxieties [*he's tearful*]. We travelled around Europe together for two months.
- At the end of this intermittent series of sessions, Luke said he felt he would be fine to go on, on his own. I endorsed that and felt both relief and elation and also sadness at finishing up our work together. He thanked me for helping him "more than you'll know".

Section C

Return to therapy (April 2015)

We had no contact until nearly four years later when Luke booked an appointment and asked to resume sessions.

Luke's relationship with Jenny is now five years old, he is fifty years old, and I am that much older, too. We are both in a different "place", very different from 2002 when we started, and different from 2011 when we finished. Luke looks the same and yet so different. He still has a shaved head, rides a motorcycle, and wears a leather jacket. But now there is a softness, a warmth, and nothing like the tense and angry energy that had been his customary disposition. Nevertheless, he continues to struggle with anger.

He and Jenny have moved back locally and are living together in his small house. While the relationship is good, Luke can feel suffocated by Jenny "always being there". He did tell her once, but he is so afraid of hurting her that he bottles it up and keeps his feelings to himself. When he said he had to work abroad for a month and she wasn't coming, she was upset. He felt racked with guilt and self-reproach—*How could he do that to her?* Once she saw him looking

---

[99] I had never heard that before! If that isn't mental health, what is?

at soft porn and he felt devastated, his heart pounding, overwhelmed with intense shame. "I do love her a lot, I want to be a safe harbour for her", he told me (reminiscent of *We Didn't Mean to go to Sea*).

He is making direct eye contact with me now and also asking how I am when he arrives for sessions. He seems genuinely interested. When I returned from a trip, he asked how it went. When I had a knee injury, he was noticeably concerned and inquired about my recovery. There was almost nothing of this in the first six years. These changes are significant. They are more than the product of our relationship being some thirteen years old now. The significance feels more to do with the quality of connection than the length of therapy. From my point of view, a capacity for empathy is part of connecting to others which, in turn, is an essential sign of mental/emotional health.

My first book was published after we'd reconvened, and I gave Luke a copy of *How Two Love: Making Your Relationship Work and Last* (2016). He had read it all by his next session and then bought five copies, to give to friends.

Luke wants to continue therapy because he feels there is a huge block in him, a reservoir of emotion filled with grief and rage. He doesn't know how to access it and knows he needs to. He wants to work on being more authentic.

We spoke more about his childhood than in previous sessions. Both his parents were miserable. It always felt like his fault. Even his brother "made him feel" that everything wrong was his fault. Now he feels responsible for Jenny's happiness. He understands that no one else's misery is really his fault, but he cannot shake the feeling. What does help is playing computer games and role-playing. He says his psyche becomes immersed in something *other* than his own past, present, or future—which gives some respite from his preoccupations with everything wrong with him, his life, the world, and this feeling of guilty responsibility.

In one dream, Luke is in a band in a club or auditorium on stage in the front row, facing the audience. There are people standing across from him including one slim teenager who is naked. He is admiring her face, her hair, then in a moment she is sitting in a chair facing forward, still naked, breasts, nipples—she is spectacularly lovely in a youthful way. Suddenly, he is overwhelmed by a feeling that he will be punished for this. And wakes feeling anxious.

I say he is suffering from a persecutory anxiety even though he hasn't done anything wrong, and Luke responds—"Are you saying I have a fear of fish?" (pause—I look puzzled). "Huh?" He continues: "a pescatory anxiety?" He smiles broadly as I can see the joke is on me. As we say in Australia, he is taking the piss, for my use of intellectual terminology. He's right. And it's funny.

Again, there is something about this. Despite his accounts of protectiveness and worry at hurting others, especially Jenny, he can make a joke at my expense knowing I won't fall apart or hold it against him.

[*At Luke's request, I have cut a paragraph here*]

He feels always on the defensive with Jenny, as in the following conversation: Jenny begins: "What's wrong …" (he feels his blood run cold, has a feeling of dread wash over him). She continues: "… with the television reception?"

I say: "This seems so much like a re-enactment of being a little boy, seeing your mother unhappy and feeling 'this must be because of me, I am the cause of her unhappiness'." Luke says: "Sounds good but I'm drawing a blank here."

The word "blank" is like a signpost pointing to dissociation. It raises questions: why can he not associate with the above idea? Why so blocked? Why is this such a no-go zone? Or have I got it completely wrong?

Luke continued: "Meanwhile I am actually the only child my mother feels turned out okay and is truly happy with the way she has been treated. I am appointed Executor of her Will and have Power of Attorney, if needed. So, I am literally responsible for her mental state if she cannot be responsible for herself. I've been sending her $200 per month for more years than I can remember, and whenever I visit her interstate, she gets wads of cash as well."

Since he was a little boy, he grabbed hold of the ideal of being good; no, more so—being a White Knight, and rescuing a damsel in distress. He has been motivated accordingly ever since, and now this gets played out with his mother, and in different ways, with his partner, Jenny.

Luke and Jenny bought a house which had an interesting effect. Luke said it gave him hope, instead of his customary feeling of waiting to die. Despite that, he said that he deeply believed there were invisible forces that would torture or kill him unless he placated them by serving:

- The system
- The family
- The authorities
- The Australian Taxation Office
- And everyone else

—by being good. Be good or be punished; he fears retribution. I suggested that he was projecting his own inner anger and aggression to some abstract entity outside of himself and then fearing an attack. He was already attacking himself anyway. This dynamic prohibits him from feeling his own desire or expressing it. Or if he does feel it, then it worries him or makes him feel bad and wrong.

Luke's anger is a consequence of not being able to express how he feels. Then, he holds it against himself. He berates himself, attacks himself, hates himself—just as we saw earlier with Clarissa. He holds it against himself, which makes him feel worse in a self-perpetuating cycle. I'm not saying this is the only reason for his anger, but it is a part of it. At the same time, Luke can express more of how he really feels to me. He also says there are things he can't share with me without worrying about hurting my feelings. I wish he would though.

If he has a memory of being less than impeccable, he has an anxiety attack (attacked again!). He feels guilty out of all proportion. This is where the phrase "sorry baby" originates, though he says it much less now. Even if the words aren't there, he will still feel a stab of misery, sadness, grief, or unhappiness—without being able to express any of it to Jenny.

It can be scarier to give up omnipotence fully and come to terms with the fact that shit just happens through no fault of your own; Luke seemed to prefer to feel guilty, though he suffered from the feeling as well.

Another dream:

> I am at a party, standing there by myself, staring at a wall, feeling miserable. Then I see Mel, you know, that girl I had a crush on years ago. She does a little dance and smiles at me. Then, she poses me a question: what is the name of the song I'm dancing to? And it cheered me up trying to answer it.

I'm impressed with this dream. He shifts from the unhappy position of isolation to cheerfulness with a girl he likes, though she rejected him in the past. There is a resilience here, a step out of solitary misery, and a sense of playfulness.

In another dream, Luke is on a sand plain, and sees an enormous Godzilla-type monster, "the original giant purple lizard". He has a weapon and fires at it. "Aaaarrrggh!!" He is perpetually in a battle with monsters and demons in himself. From there he went right on to speak about feeling angry with Jenny. He said he would never abuse her. I said: "You can be angry without being abusive." From there, as if anger with Jenny segued seamlessly to anger at his brother, he said that his brother visited, and he found him less offensive than ever before. He still feels wary but not nearly so charged or threatened. I am reminded that it was issues regarding Luke's brother that brought him to therapy initially, though he featured as a subject in relatively few sessions.

Despite the presence of residual painful and conflicted feelings, Luke said at this point that I had helped him a great deal and he greatly appreciated it. His expression felt genuine and authentic, and touched me. We had been going a long time and been through much together. Again, there was a feeling of connection, of endowing the therapy process with value, and of gratitude—qualities that are essential parts of meaningful living.

The next session began with Luke smiling at me as he entered the room—"Hi! How are you?" There is more warmth here than ever before. He seems pleased to see me and happy to be here; indeed, he is positively animated—this is just so different. This is not the "Hi! How are you?" that we're asked at the checkout of the supermarket, with a mechanical politeness and false familiarity born of training. This is a greeting between two people who mean something to each other.

I realise Luke is not "completely well" after all this therapy. Who is completely well? Yet, I do see significant development alongside his many issues. This is exactly where polarising illness and wellness in a binary opposition makes no sense at all. Each position disavows what is significant in the other position. He is well in some ways and not in others, sometimes more than others. It varies. At the very least, he has a possibility of happiness, connection, sexual intimacy, companionship, and meaningfulness, even if a truly peaceful mental state remains somewhat remote.

I was five minutes late for the next session with Luke. In the past he would have looked disapproving if I kept him waiting for two minutes, but this day, he was relaxed and said not to worry about it. He went on: "I've been riding to work beating myself up in my mind for not loving better, more fully, more freely than I have been. I realised it was the guilt I carry with me all the time that prevents me." I said: "Maybe that is the point. Your guilt isn't about something you've done or even would like to do but guilt functions to protect you from the vulnerability of really opening your heart and loving more fully and freely." Luke said: "Maybe."

We went on to speak of the difficulty of being fully loving which privileges the interests of the other and being fully sexual which privileges the interests of oneself. Me: "Of course, you can derive gratification from giving love just as you can from giving pleasure in sex. It doesn't have to be a one-way strcct." Hc said it is hard to even allow himself to feel desire. He went on but in a different direction: "I did raise my voice angrily at Jenny, and I have to say, she took it well. I really have to rise above the terror of offending her."

Luke: I have always wanted to be with a woman that could be a "confident comforter" to me, someone who would hold me and allow me to lie on her breast.

Me: Tell her.

Luke: I don't want to impose, she has so much of her own "stuff" to deal with.

Me: Has it occurred to you that she might like it? I don't know how she'll take that or how she'll feel about it. But it seems to me that she might just feel a little better about her own stuff if she can be of value and help you with yours.

Luke: Some of my resentment is from feeling that I can't expect too much from her because of all she has to deal with, mainly from her own history.

Me: Tell her that.

Luke: Maybe … [*Pause*] She is very loving at the moment, but I feel afraid I will step on a mine that explodes. I need to get to this deep reservoir of guilt and anxiety that comes from very early. Sometimes, I feel split between a sexually impotent nice guy and a violent/aggressive bloke who forces his sexual needs on a woman.

Me: The middle ground is elusive. Of course, you can allow your needs to be expressed without having to be violent or aggressive or imposing them.

Luke: You know, I never felt a natural love for my mother, but I felt like I had to exhibit it. I felt forced to choose between hurting her or betraying myself by acting inauthentically. I am carrying so much anger toward women. I think I missed out on a ton of sex when I was younger because of it.

Me: So, you became a nice guy, a protector and saviour-rescuer as a young man and went passive and distant instead of acting on the anger.

A month passed. When Luke came in next, he told me he had proposed to Jenny, and she jumped at it. "Amazing!" I exclaimed delightedly. They will marry in three or four months. I remembered all the years, more than ten, that Luke had no partners at all. He said he felt a bit sad not to feel more romantic about it, but he said that he walked out of their new home the other day while listening to a song and felt content about where his life was. He imagined himself as a younger man, projecting into the future and seeing himself as he is right now. He felt comforted by that. He felt a sense of surrender to accepting the person he is. And then: "Apart from my interior landscape of guilt and misery, and sometimes the gigantic storm clouds of anger, I'm doing okay."

The next month he was working abroad, but when he returned, he told me that he had been playing a lot of badminton there, it was so much fun. It was even more fun when they got drunk and played drunken badminton. After one insane rally everyone wound up falling on the ground in unison, rolling around, and laughing hysterically. It was hilarious.

He continued in a more serious vein: "Sometimes I feel like I am the guy who was supposed to solve the problem of my mother's unhappiness and my father's unhappiness. Sometimes, my love for Jenny feels a little clinical, like I'm not really feeling what I'm supposed to be feeling, even though I appear to be."

Me: Like for your mother.
Luke: Yes, then I remembered that one of the criticisms that my father levelled against my mother was that her love for us kids was clinical. She worked as a nurse. She did all the practical things well, but mechanically, her emotional involvement was lacking. The only times she was more relaxed in her feelings was when she'd been drinking.
Me: Wow! I've never heard that before.
Luke: Sometimes I feel like I've answered the question of the meaning of life without any reference to my own desire. I'm going out to the kitchen to make myself a cup of tea as an expression of my desire at this moment.

Luke had never walked out of the room in the middle of a session before. When he returned, he said: I can see that my guilt is an expression of concern for other people. I actually do like looking after people. It's just that I feel that if I'm not actively being good, I'm bad.

Me: Not every thought or action is a moral issue. There is another option, a third possibility.
Luke: What's that?
Me: It's the middle zone of desire, it is perfectly possible to want something for yourself and for that to be neither good nor bad, not compromising to anyone else.
Luke: What is the word for the opposite of ontological insecurity?
Me: Huh? [*I couldn't see the relevance*]
Luke: Being.

Two months have passed since Luke's last appointment. The interval between sessions is getting longer. They are struggling financially and needing to be careful with spending on non-essentials. And they had a small wedding to pay for. Luke and Jenny married on the beach. He said it was wonderful and thanked me for the card I sent. I had been thinking of them, being very aware of the timing of these events. It felt beautifully symbolic to me, and I felt celebratory hearing about it. Luke was so happy as he described the event. I felt emotional hearing Luke *that* happy.

He went on to say that his mother was in hospital with pneumonia—he felt miserable about that—he helped organise getting her apartment cleaned. "You could scrape the nicotine off the walls with a knife!" And his father had fallen and hurt his shoulder. Both parents are in their eighties now.

From there, he spoke about a recent role-playing event. Here, Luke was more animated, more excited, more energised than I've ever seen him. He'd given his mate an instruction in the game and his friend did the opposite—which had consequences for them. Luke was ENRAGED! He was fully expressing it in my room though he said he felt constrained to express it at the time.

As he left, I said: "Hey, congratulations again on getting married, I'm really happy about it." Luke lit up, smiled broadly, looked me in the eyes, and shook my hand appreciatively. I felt we were truly connected.

In the next session two months on, Luke said the same thing happened in role-playing. This time, instead of feeling enraged, he laughed and felt a sense of "defeatist-acceptance". Later, he did confront his friend about it but gently. His friend didn't take it well and said he would never play again. Then he got over it and did play and followed directions—which worked better. I felt he had managed his own emotions well and his communication was effective and said so.

Two months later (2018)

Luke: We need to talk about anger. Jenny wants me to get angry. Now I'm feeling guilty for not getting angry. Then I feel angry because I'm feeling guilty.

Me: It sounds like you're trying to keep yourself safe, but it's not safe to be feeling so angry and guilty and miserable.

Luke: You're right in that it prevents me from an authentic enjoyment of my life. But otherwise, you're wrong. [*Smiles, looking pleased at having trumped me. Then he reports a dream*] I'm sitting on a chair by a doorway, drinking tea. A woman appears and asks "Would you like a different sort of milk?" Then, she pops a breast in my mouth and squeezes out a drop of milk. It was nice.

Me: [I look inquisitive. *He is used to my asking what he thinks dreams mean*]

Luke: Hmm, the milk of human kindness, somehow the world can be nourishing.

Me: I wonder if milk signifies motherly love? I think you find it hard to believe that love can be given to you from a woman without your having to give something in return, having to pay for it in a sense, or do something, be heroic. It is as if there is something required of you, just being, being you seems not enough to be loved. I wonder if your guilt arises simply from your being?[100]

---

[100] This can be called existential or ontological guilt—a feeling of guilt that arises from your being and not anything done or even intended—a condition far more common, in my experience, than generally recognised.

Luke: I feel near to crying. [*Pause*] What you said last time about a third possibility other than good or bad has helped. [*Then, he offers me a chocolate-coated liquorice*]

Me: Thanks! Yum!

Luke: I saw the latest *Star Wars*. It made me so angry, so furious, I can't tell you. [*Then he gets animated again, like before when he was enraged about the role-playing. He is fully going off now*] Anger leads to hate. And hate is the gateway to the dark side.

Me: You know, you don't have to be a Jedi …

Meaning-fullness (2018)

The aim of this book is to explore where meaning comes from, what to do about a lack of meaningful living, and to make life worth living where it isn't already. This is the undergirding of mental health, though it is missing from the medical model insofar as it is followed by psychology and psychiatry.

Experience of therapy over time shows there are "things" that change and "things" that do not change. Whether or not those "things" that have not changed *can* change remains open. Not everything can or does.[101] Where something does not change or changes very little, then your relation to that issue becomes paramount. If you can come to terms (in the double sense, as we've indicated about symbolisation) then the consequence of the issue is mitigated, even if the issue stands relatively unchanged.

With Luke, some "things" have changed and other "things" not—it might be tempting to say: "Given that, how is so much therapy justified?" A professional relationship is a living, breathing, evolving "thing". It is not like buying a car that depreciates in value over time. Quite the opposite. Those who have been through psychotherapy know its value grows for them long after sessions have finished.

It's hard to assess what has changed for Luke or how much. Many of the "changes" are either intangible or highly subjective. On that note, I don't think any objective measure would produce a more meaningful statement than I can give from my own subjective experience and the corresponding descriptions.

I find him a warm person now, also mainly calm, unlike at the beginning. He can have peaceful moods and a more balanced disposition. He is often animated and alive; his voice is expressive with feelings not in evidence at the outset. He is engaged in our exchanges and can be playful and light-hearted. He can get angry and bring a sense of regulated hate to that which he objects to. And he can act on his passion for the environment, directly within the limits of his reach. He is fully sexual, loves his wife, who loves him, wrestles with the issues between

---

[101] On this point, I have often said to patients "I would have liked to be taller but never will be" as an example of something that cannot change, it must be lived with and just as well to come to terms with it. Accept it. Then, let it go. However, in 2014, I had bilateral knee replacement surgery and my legs were straightened in the process. Ironically, I gained nearly two inches in height—contrary to the very example I used of what cannot change, had!

them and has built a life full of meaning. When I think back to where he was when we started, I feel celebratory—this was work worth doing—despite the long periods of feeling we were wandering through a desert without an oasis in view.

Most therapists can parade examples of their clinical work where dramatic improvements occur sometimes in a short time. We all love those cases. You feel like a genius, and the patient and often their associates, regard you as a rock-star therapist. However, most therapy works incrementally over time, if by "works" we mean relief of suffering and lasting development.

The work with Luke has not been easy. Yet, it has become easier, lighter, and more enjoyable. I look forward to seeing him and the feeling is mutual. This is the heart of meaning-fullness.

Unscientific postscript

I am indulging in a private joke here, borrowing from the title of Kierkegaard's[102] major work (1941) which attacks Hegel's science of logic and objectivism (1910). Hegel's work was a kind of hyper-rationality that shares some similarities with the presuppositions of mainstream psychology, psychiatry, general medicine, and other mental health practices. *Meaning-Fullness* is in direct contradistinction and presents an alternative view.

As the long case of Luke has largely summarised the main points of this book and contextualised them clinically in an example of developmental psychotherapy, what follows are concluding and further summary thoughts.

The problem with over emphasising logic and rationality is that it lacks heart. Therapeutic practice must not lose heart or mind if promoting mental health. This harks back to my work in training therapists when I spoke of therapy as the practice of thoughtfulness and compassion.

Mental health practices are now so full of techniques, strategies, advice, medications, new age practices, "answers" and "solutions" that patients now come requesting them, indeed sometimes demanding them, and can become aggrieved if they are not provided.

---

[102] Kierkegaard is a master of irony, and the great irony of *Concluding Unscientific Postscript* is that it is a postscript to his earlier work *Philosophical Fragments* but roughly two or three times longer, so hardly a postscript.

> The question *How to stop mental suffering?*
> doesn't have a set answer.
> It is not a problem for which a known solution exists.
> You are not a broken machine that needs repair.
> Mental pain is not a bodily injury to be treated as such.
> Mental illness is usually not a disease like other diseases.

It is easy to be confused. You can feel wounded, damaged, broken, or ill—indeed, these metaphors may fit your experience—but that does not mean your suffering is the same as a physical condition where the same metaphors apply.

The development aimed for through psychotherapy involves cultivating capacities of thinking for yourself, generating a sense of agency, knowing your desire, and feeling the fullest possible range of emotions, integrated with, and connected to, what is happening, as it happens. It is not about being happy, chirpy, and positive every day—it's not wrong if you are—but positivity is not all there is to "real life". What real life *means* varies for each of us. What matters is that it means *something*.

There is how you feel and what happens to you. Sometimes, how you feel is directly correlated with what happens and sometimes not. Ideally, I think it is desirable to dwell in a largely neutral zone, neither especially "up" nor "down" in mood or disposition. When "things" happen in the course of a day, when, say, an important event goes for you or against you, let's respond to that. If someone says something a little snide, maybe it bothers you, or not. It's okay either way. If there is loss, then grieve it by processing how it feels and what that means. If there is injustice, feel angry or outraged. If there is love, then take it in, feel loved. And if a two-year-old is excited to see you, runs into your open arms, and nuzzles into the nape of your neck as you pick them up, feel the full intensity of joy that brings.

Throughout this "journey", I have tried to focus my binoculars of thought to bring into view the meaning of mental health beyond what the reference books, Google, or Wikipedia has to offer.

Overview

The broad field of mental health is in crisis and getting worse. We ask: why, when there has never been so much psychology and psychiatry available? The over-medicalisation of mental unwellness begins to point to an answer. I am not saying we must throw it out completely. The emphasis is wrong. It leads us to view mental/emotional suffering as a bodily imbalance, disorder, or condition. Obviously, there are correlations between body and mind. Viewing the body as the source or cause is a mistake and leads us down limited pathways or dead ends, with some exceptions. In most cases, there is no scientific evidence for it—contrary to popular opinion. The body and mind are then split as if two separate entities.

There is a confusion around what mental unwellness means that arises out of the polarisation and opposition of concepts of health and illness. At what point does feeling down or low mood become a diagnosable mental disorder? The rating scales and questionnaires do not provide an objective answer or agree with each other. Besides, such mental states are often highly variable. People do get stuck in states like depression that can last for months or years. Depression can become entrenched and unmovable, immutable. I have never seen a single patient in forty-five years of practice where we could not uncover an underlying reason for their depression. The point here is not that understanding miraculously relieves depression. Sometimes, understanding does help, sometimes not. The important point is that depression, like all mental suffering, is *meaningful*.

When we reach to the meaning of mental/emotional pain, we open the possibility of a conversation about it. Such conversations make a difference, especially if to the point, as psychotherapy needs to be. The theoretical portion of this book argues that an understanding of early childhood development and its vicissitudes, challenges, and limits, positions therapists to work towards releasing emotional development where it has not been seen through. Such development involves the growth of capacities for affective living; that is, feeling the fullest possible intensity of your feelings, resilience, ability to cope with stress and distress, a sense of separateness and relatedness, identity, and the ability to act as an agent on your own behalf—proactively, in your own best interest. Even the capacity to let yourself know what is in your best interest, or not, makes a world of difference. Knowing what you want, how you feel, the limits and boundaries of your interactions with others, keeping yourself safe, cultivating intuition, erotic experience, and healthy sexuality, and not least, the capacity to love and receive love, are all examples. Finding your way, a quiet mind and relaxed body, being at peace with yourself, care, and empathy for others, listening out for what calls you to speak or act according to your own authentic true values—are further examples. We should not omit financial health, passing socially, paying bills, the ability to live without excessive money worries or toxic debt; these are vital elements of mental health, especially as conditions worsen. What does mental health mean to you?

What research can add is somewhat questionable as mental health is such a personal and individual consideration. Research tends to produce statistical averages and generalities. These can be useful. There are ways we are all the same and I am not against making the most of what research has to offer. Notwithstanding my criticisms, there are some excellent and skilled researchers who produce useful studies, largely free from bias or vested interests. I am just deeply sceptical of the emphasis placed on the need for research, and the difficulty of how to tell the difference between scrupulous and unscrupulous research.

When we speak of research, psychology, psychiatry, psychotherapy, development, mental illness, and a host of other terms, we are not referring to one unified, singular concept. This makes discussions, such as those in this book, difficult. There is a huge range of differences in every category. Descriptors like *psychotherapist* are used differently by different professionals, which makes a hot mess for the public trying to make sense out of the mental health professions. That is just it, it doesn't make any sense. I am trying to bring sense—meaning—to a highly disordered situation. It would probably take ten lifetimes to make a dent.

The question *What makes life worth living?* is not usually part of mental health practices, and that includes psychotherapy practices. Some people never need to ask this question. Winnicott notes the difference between genuine development and a "successful analysis", where the mental disorder or issues that brought the patient were resolved, but they still have no reason for living. When this existential question remains at issue—it is not an illness though it may function like one—it must no longer be ignored if we are to improve the mental health of the community and ourselves as individuals.

The question doesn't have to have an answer or a reason. To be frank, I myself don't have a *reason* for living. I don't feel the lack of one either. It is not an issue, and it doesn't have to be. For myself, I am given this life to live; I find myself in this position with this body and mind and functional resources, for better and worse. From here, the *I am* position, I look outside myself at the world and ask what is needed. What I see is a world that is fucked, and getting "fuckeder", and one that is FULL of suffering but not FULL of meaning.

If I could, the first thing I would redress is the segregation of wealth in the hands of a ridiculous minority and the deprivation of it from the masses. This is a monstrous global crime of our own making and a massive contributor to mental suffering, physical illness, and literal crime. I should have said more on this earlier, but it needs a whole book, if not a library, to do the subject justice. I don't know what I can do about that. I feel powerless in the face of this macro-socio-economic catastrophe of late capitalism. So, I work—as much as I can—small scale: one person or couple or family group at a time, one day at a time, one session at a time. Like ripples in a pond, I believe that the therapeutic benefits flow out to my patients, then to their significant others and their significant others and so on. As Popeye says, *I am what I am*. I am a therapist, teacher, writer, husband, father, grandfather, friend. That's it. But it's not about me, it's about you. Who are you?

The existential vacuum is missing in action in mental health practices. Try going to a professional person and saying "I feel empty inside" and see what happens. Blank stares, change the subject, deep-breathing techniques suggested—"You just need a good root, mate" (one patient said he was actually told this by a mental health professional! "Root" is Australian vernacular for "screw", "bonk", "fuck", or simply "sex"). Or we can always blame your brain or your mother. Not good enough! *Meaning-Fullness* is an alternative mental health approach that includes the profound questions of existence without pretending to have all the answers.

The inclusion of an understanding of language in its broadest sense is vital for our mental health practices and for growing a capacity for meaning-making in our lives. Language as intentional, rather than referential, points to considerations of what people mean by what they say. Our reliance upon reference books such as DSM to categorise mental disorders is a gross mistake and again, follows a medical perspective to treatments of variable efficacy that lack meaning or context. The reference point is meaning, not diagnosis. The best use of diagnosis I know, and one that employs an understanding of character organisation in the service of psychotherapeutic clinical process is Nancy McWilliams' *Psychoanalytic Diagnosis* (2011). I taught this text to psychotherapists and psychiatry registrars to good effect because its use of diagnosis was not confined to a narrow definition of mental disorder, collections of "symptoms" or "syndromes". Diagnosis can be useful if it isn't too reductive but does not replace understanding what a patient means by what they say or don't say. Nothing does. Now, there is also the second edition of the *Psychodynamic Diagnostic Manual* (Lingiardi & McWilliams, 2017)[103] which is much improved and bridges the gap between the DSM and clinical complexity.

Generally, I find patients are urgent to get out of the state they're in—understandably if it is painful. Often the methods employed to "get out of it" compound the issue, defer, or avoid it. This strategy of putting it off until later is not effective and often brings "side-effects", destructive consequences, or a kind of energy drain, distance from the issue, at worst—a deadening. Symbolisation points in the opposite direction. It refers to a coming to terms with what needs to be addressed. It is sitting in it, being with yourself—even if that involves suffering—and going through what must be gone through, not more and not less. It helps to address issues with another person who cares and understands. It probably won't get far if done through intellectualisation, rationalisation, scientism, psychologising, or split-off explanations. Split-off from what? Abstract theoretical explanations miss the body, lack heart and mind, and thus miss the point. They also often miss the situation itself in the present or the historical context of the past. Hence, embodied symbolisation is the term I use for meaningful reflections and discussions on the issue that bears down upon you. Psychotherapy with both heartfulness + mindfulness = meaning-fullness.

Within the limits of human frailty, the ideal vehicle for mental and emotional (and physical) development is a secure attachment with someone positively disposed to attend to your needs. This is the case for infants, small children, larger and older children, teenagers, young adults, and everyone else, from birth through to senescence. There is no age limit for development. Emotional and spiritual development differs from physical development. We can witness a child's physical growth, we notice progress, we can measure their height against the wall, we detect spurts of growth and periods of recess. Emotional and spiritual growth are harder to detect, impossible to measure, and exist in a metaphysical realm. Like electricity, it is hard to identify exactly what it is, but we can see what it does, its effects. Sometimes, people notice

---

[103] It has separate sections for infancy, childhood, adolescence, adulthood, and old age and emphasises developmental processes in its "Mental Functions" axis. The *PDM* is a way of thinking about people for purposes of clinical understanding and emphasises inference, dimensionality, context, and meaning. It is the first major classification system to include a section on issues of the elderly.

something has changed. One patient came with a phobia about driving. We got to the bottom of it in one session; she'd had an accident through no fault of her own years ago. She was more frightened by it than injured. The memory of it haunted her, what could have happened, but its fearfulness evaporated as we separated out past from present, and she was fine to drive after that. This was a positive change and immediate benefit. Development is usually more subtle, harder to assess, resistant to definition, and typically takes time. It can happen in an instant, a flash of insight, an epiphany, a realisation—but it can take quite a lot of therapeutic work to arrive at that instant. An example of a woman in her mid-twenties comes to mind:

> She was angry at her parents. She spoke a great deal about how irresponsible they had been in her childhood. They were hippies, inherited money, lived a middle-class life but were often stoned, forgot to collect her from school or pack a lunch for her. And so on. We spoke about it over many sessions.
>
> About a year later she reported she no longer felt angry. She realised her parents did the best they could; they probably weren't ready to have children at a young age and they were a product of their culture at the time. Her relationship with both parents improved once she stopped holding something against them.

This is a simple example of development. My patient had "grown up", come to terms with aspects of her history, and became able to integrate them into her field of experience. Carrying anger and resentment can otherwise land you with a diagnosis of a mental disorder (when nothing is causing it in the present). Her reflections and our discussion about them made a tangible difference. Although she couldn't change her history, its effect upon her changed radically.

I could have just said "Your parents did the best they could, and you need to come to terms with that." I could see that. "You wanted your parents to be more grown up than they were and look after you more responsibly. That's not unreasonable but it just wasn't the reality of your childhood." I didn't say that. My position was primarily to validate her feelings while gently challenging some of her assertions. She came to her own realisations in her own time. The benefit is characterological change that lasts. She has matured and so feels resolved about the past.

The emphasis on short-term outcomes pre-empts lasting development. Patients may feel better initially after sessions but nothing has really changed. Then, they're back in six months or a year (or less!). I see this frequently in mental health practices. Patients' needs become a revolving door because they have not been properly attended to in the first place.

There is a saying from trauma-informed therapy: *Slower is faster*. So simple. And true. It runs counter to the drive for short-term results and economic savings, making mental health care more affordable from a governmental point of view. The way to make mental health care cost less is to help patients enough so they don't have to keep coming back again and again. Short-termism is a false economy, though it is wonderful—occasionally—when someone too afraid to drive turns that around in a single session.

I have spoken a lot about play. Speaking for myself, when I approach my clinical work as play, without trivialising it in the slightest, it is less exhausting, taxing, onerous, or disturbing, it creates less of a psychic load for me to carry through my days and nights. I would say the same thing about approaching the living of my personal life as play. Everything feels easier, though I hold the same commitments and responsibilities. It lightens and enlightens.

I have certainly been subject to the cultural injunction to work as productively as possible. I had cancer in 1996, almost certainly a direct consequence of overwork and stress. At first, it looked like "game-over" (and you don't get extra "lives" in this one). Was it necessary to overwork to that degree? It felt like it at the time. With hindsight, it wasn't. As a culture, we are working ourselves to death, prematurely. We are ageing faster than we need to, even if some are living longer. This is not the same as development. I see people concerned about their financial security and for good reason. What are they doing about that? Working harder, for longer. You can build a secure future of wealth and die before you get there. We never really consider that or believe it. Thus, the value of an illusion—it is motivating—but also brings the corresponding inverse need for disillusion, or consequences follow.

The reality is you are better off living below your means than beyond them (I'm such a bad example, still trying to learn this). Productivity is desirable but needs to be brought into balance with doing things of value for their own sake and accepting that our total psycho-physiological systems need down-time and rest.

We spoke about living authentically and destroying projections, which include agendas, demands, needs, and pressure both from others to do or be what they want, and in yourself towards others. The contradiction that destroying the object of your desire leaves you more likely to get what you want is one of the strange conundrums of living. If you leave space—potential space—the other can meet you at the site of your desire without being positioned by you, free from manipulation or pressure. The potential space allows (the possibility of) their desire meeting yours.

Potential space is a difficult concept but a valuable one. It is a space where development happens, where capacities can be expanded, and where personal growth unfolds. In the example of the small child whose mother leaves the room to answer the front door, the child can get anxious about being left alone or get involved with something of interest. Potential space affords an opportunity to develop a capacity to be alone and feel okay. It is easy to extrapolate to adult experience.

If alone, potential space affords an opportunity to sit in the discomfort zone of your own feelings. They won't kill you. If you can bear your own feelings, if you can go through what there is to be gone through, then you may find there is so much to play with, to interest and engage, to enjoy, even have fun. Your capacities have the possibility of growth and development in this open space of potential. What can you make of it? Is there something to be found? Can you create something?

If you can be alone, and remain comfortable and functional, you are in a better position to be in a relationship that works.

When we come to the professional relationship, we are at the centrepiece of the psychotherapeutic process. I gave examples, though really every case is its own unique example. No relationship is the same as any other. Novice therapists tend to be focused on being "good" therapists, like the psychiatry registrar who was so concerned about breaking rules, he didn't think about what it meant that his patient gave her baby to him to hold. Similarly, I have one parent after another concerned about their parenting. Are they doing it right? Are they a good parent? Are they good-enough? Without detracting from the importance of these concerns, when you realise that both parenting and therapy revolve around a relationship, it becomes less about doing it right or being good at it. The focus becomes more about what happens between you, the meaning of your interactions. Whether or not the patient was saying in an indirect symbolic way *You can hold the baby part of myself in therapy*, as I suggested to the registrar, is open to interpretation. There can be little doubt this was a gesture of trust that speaks volumes to me about the quality of their interactions over three sessions. To me, the registrar understood little about psychotherapy. He'd had some training and some reading behind him. He was really fumbling about in the dark. His personality, however, was well suited to therapy. He was reliable, attentive, caring, responsive, connected, and gentle. He was soft-spoken and unthreatening. The forty sessions of the "long-case" went well, and indeed this patient was relieved of much anxiety, reduced conflict with her parents, improved relationship issues with her partner, and grew into a more confident mum. She also made progress towards a higher education degree. As the registrar became more comfortably situated in the relationship with the patient, the therapy worked better.

I wouldn't like to imply that anyone with the right personality can just put up a shingle, call themselves a psychotherapist, and start practising without training. Some of my trainees, however, who were not university-educated but had spent twenty years raising children, or working as hairdressers, taxi drivers, and bar tenders, turned out to be better psychotherapists than some with higher education degrees. Why? The ones with degrees were generally better at study. The others had spent their time listening to people, trying to understand them, hearing their stories, and attending to expressions of pain, loss, or sorrow. Who would you rather consult, someone knowledgeable or someone understanding?

Lastly, the great irony of transformation: it is the seeking, the striving, the longing and yearning to be more, better, different, that prevents you being where you are, grounded in yourself. Being there, where you are, is the condition of the possibility of personal growth. Transformation comes in all shapes and forms, but there is literally nothing outside of yourself that can make you more of yourself. Think about it. It doesn't make sense. If I won the Lottery, sure it would relieve financial pressure, but I would still have the messed-up psychology around money where I spend too much, where I am overly generous and sometimes get rid of money I cannot afford to dispense with (such as risky investments). The likelihood is: all of that could be exponentially worse if I had more money, and still harboured a fantasy of being Father Christmas.

> The transformation you seek is
> freedom from the need to be transformed.

One woman who weighed ninety kilos said she was tired of having no suiters. She had her stomach stapled and indeed lost literally half her weight. I met her as a forty-five-kilo woman. She told me she had a queue of male admirers wanting to go out with her. She enjoyed the attention and duly registered the extreme shift in attitude, but now she deeply resented the fact that men found her desirable whereas they didn't before. Now that she had engineered men to desire her, she didn't desire them. In fact, she resented their admiration because *She was the same person!*

> The surprising irony of development:
> coming to terms with what is
> sets you free to develop.

It may seem like a contradiction that this text espouses the need and the value of emotional development, implying a forward movement. Then, I turn around and say *Be yourself* and *You don't need to strive after anything that promises transformation.* The difference here is that emotional development sometimes happens organically, and other times needs the focused work of psychotherapy when it has stalled. Anyone who has experienced this will understand that you don't have to chase development. You don't have to pursue mental health. You don't have to discover some elusive data to be yourself or to reformat yourself. Development is what happens to you when you stop chasing it and attend to what needs attention. As that happens, you can see it is the necessary precondition to find and create meaning, to live a life of meaning-fullness.

THE END

References

A Two-Year Old goes to Hospital (1952). James Robertson. Tavistock Clinic and Concord Media.

Bachelard, G. (1964). *The Psychoanalysis of Fire*. Boston: Beacon Press.

Bromberg, P. (1998). *Standing in the Spaces: Essays on Clinical Process, Trauma and Dissociation*. Hillsdale, NJ: Analytic.

Castonguay, L. G., & Muran, C. (2015). Fostering collaboration between researchers and clinicians through building practice-oriented research: An introduction. *Psychotherapy Research*, *25*(1): 1–5. https://doi.org/10.1080/10503307.2014.966348

Castonguay, L. G., Youn, S. J., Xiao, H., Muran, C., & Barber, J. P. (2015). Building clinician-researcher partnerships: Lessons from diverse natural settings and practice-oriented initiatives. *Psychotherapy Research*, *25*(1): 116–184. https://doi.org/10.1080/10503307.2014.973923

Castonguay, L. G., Constantino, M. J., & Beutler, L. E. (Eds.) (2019). *Principles of Change: How Psychotherapists Implement Research in Practice*. New York: Oxford University.

Chapman, G. (1992). *The 5 Love Languages: The Secret to a Love that Lasts*. Chicago: Northfield.

Cooper, S. H. (2021). Donald Winnicott and Stephen Mitchell's Developmental Tilt Hypothesis Reconsidered. *Psychoanalytic Dialogues*, *31*(3): 355–370.

Csikszentmihalyi, M. (1990). *Flow: The Psychology of Optimal Experience*. New York: Harper & Row.

Dalal, F. (2018). *CBT: The Cognitive Behavioural Tsunami—Managerialism, Politics, and the Corruptions of Science*. New York: Routledge.

DSM-5. *Diagnostic and Statistical Manual of Mental Disorders*. (2013). Arlington, VA: American Psychiatric Association.

Eigen, M. (1999). The Area of Faith in Winnicott, Lacan and Bion. In: S. A Mitchell & L. Aron, (Eds.), *Relational Psychoanalysis: The Emergence of a Tradition* (pp. 1–37). Hillsdale, NJ: Analytic.

Fonagy, P., Luyten, P., Allison, E., & Campbell, C. (2019). Mentalizing, epistemic trust and the phenomenology of psychotherapy. University College London eprint. https://discovery.ucl.ac.uk/id/eprint/10076243/1/Fonagy_Mentalising%20and%20phenomenology_revised.pdf

Fonagy, P., Gergely, G., Jurist, E., & Target, M. (2004). *Affect Regulation, Mentalization and the Development of the Self.* New York: Other Press.

Frankl, V. E. (2014). *Man's Search for Meaning.* Boston: Beacon.

Frankl, V. E. (1970). *The Will to Meaning: Foundations and Applications of Logotherapy.* New York: Meridian.

Frankl, V. E. (1986). *The Doctor and the Soul: From Psychotherapy to Logotherapy.* New York: Vintage.

Furman, E. (1982). Mothers Have to Be There to Be Left. *The Psychoanalytic Study of the Child, 37*: 15–28.

Gadamer, H-G. (1975). *Truth and Method.* London: Sheed and Ward.

Ghent, E. (1990). Masochism, Submission, Surrender: Masochism as a Perversion of Surrender. In: S. Mitchell & L. Aron (Eds.), *Relational Psychoanalysis: The Emergence of a Tradition* (pp. 211–242). NJ: Analytic, 1999.

Goleman, D. (1985). *Vital Lies, Simple Truths: The Psychology of Self-Deception.* New York: Simon & Schuster.

Green, A. (1986). The Dead Mother. In: *On Private Madness* (pp. 142–173). London: Hogarth.

Heaton, J. M. (2006). From Anti-psychiatry to Critical Psychiatry. In: D. B. Double (Ed.), *Critical Psychiatry: The Limits of Madness* (pp. 41–60). Basingstoke, Hampshire: Palgrave Macmillan.

Heaton, J. M. (2010a). *The Talking Cure: Wittgenstein's Therapeutic Method for Psychotherapy.* Basingstoke, Hampshire: Palgrave McMillan.

Heaton, J. M. (2010b). *The Talking Cure: Wittgenstein on Language as Bewitchment and Clarity.* Basingstoke, Hampshire: Palgrave Macmillan.

Heaton, J. M. (2014). *Wittgenstein and Psychotherapy, from Paradox to Wonder.* Basingstoke, Hampshire: Palgrave Macmillan.[104]

Hegel, G. W. F. (1910). *The Phenomenology of Mind.* London: Macmillan.

Heidegger, M. (1962). *Being and Time.* Oxford: Basil Blackwell.

Herman, J. (1992). *Trauma and Recovery: The Aftermath of Violence—From Domestic Abuse to Political Terror.* New York: Basic.

Huizinga, J. (1970). *Homo Ludens: A Study of the Play-Element in Culture.* London: Paladin.

Huizinga, J. (2006). Nature and Significance of Play as a Cultural Phenomenon. In: K. Salen & E. Zimmerman (Eds.), *The Games Design Reader, A Rules of Play Anthology* (pp. 96–121). Cambridge, MA: MIT.

Insel, T. (2013, January). Toward a New Understanding of Mental Illness. Caltech: TEDx. https://www.ted.com/talks/thomas_insel_toward_a_new_understanding_of_mental_illness?language=en

Jung, C. G. (1933). *Modern Man in Search of a Soul.* New York: Harcourt, Brace & World.

Jung, C. G. (1963). *Memories, Dreams, Reflections.* New York: Pantheon.

---

[104] Although not cited in the text, this book has been an important source.

Kawa, S., & Giordano, J. (2012). A Brief Historicity of the *Diagnostic and Statistical Manual of Mental Disorders*: Issues and Implications for the Future of Psychiatric Canon and Practice. *Philosophy, Ethics and Humanities in Medicine, 7*: 2. https://doi.org/10.1186/1747-5341-7-2

Kezelman, C., & Stavropoulos, P. (2102). *The Last Frontier: Practice Guidelines for Treatment of Complex Trauma and Trauma Informed Care and Service Delivery*. Sydney: Blue Knot Foundation. https://www.blueknot.org.au/

Kezelman, C., & Stavropoulos, P. (2019). *Practice Guidelines for Clinical Treatment of Complex Trauma: Empowering Recovery from Complex Trauma*. Sydney: Blue Knot Foundation. https://www.blueknot.org.au/

Kierkegaard, S. (1941). *Concluding Unscientific Postscript*. Princeton, NJ: Princeton University Press.

Krupnick, J. L., Sotsky, S. M., Simmens, S., Moyer, J., Elkin, I., Watkins, J., & Pilkonis, P. A. (1996). The Role of the Therapeutic Alliance in Psychotherapy and Pharmacotherapy Outcome: Findings in the National Institute of Mental Health Treatment of Depression Collaborative Research Program. *Journal of Consulting and Clinical Psychology, 64*(3): 537.

Laing, R. D. (1965). *The Divided Self: An Existential Study in Sanity and Madness*. Harmondsworth, Middlesex: Penguin.

Levinas, E. (1969). *Totality and Infinity: An Essay on Exteriority*. Pittsburgh: Duquesne University.

Life is Beautiful (1997). Directed by Roberto Benigni. Melampo Cinematografica.

Lingiardi, V., & McWilliams, N. (2017). *Psychodynamic Diagnostic Manual 2nd Edition*. New York: Guilford.

McWilliams, N. (2004). *Psychoanalytic Psychotherapy: A Practitioner's Guide*. New York: Guilford.

McWilliams, N. (2011). *Psychoanalytic Diagnosis: Understanding Personality Structure in the Clinical Process*. New York: Guilford.

McWilliams, N. (2017). Integrative Research for Integrative Practice: A Plea for Respectful Collaboration Across Clinician and Researcher Roles. *Journal of Psychotherapy Integration, 27*(3): 283–195. http://dx.doi.org/10.1037/int0000054

Merleau-Ponty, M. (1962). *The Phenomenology of Perception*. London: Routledge & Kegan Paul.

Mitchell, S. A. (1984). Object Relations Theories and the Developmental Tilt. *Contemporary Psychoanalysis, 20*(4): 473–499. https://doi.org/10.1080/00107530.1984.10745749

Moland, L. L. (2021). Friedrich Schiller. In: E. N. Zalta (Ed.), *The Stanford Encyclopedia of Philosophy*. https://plato.stanford.edu/archives/sum2021/entries/schiller/

Moncrieff, J. (2011). The Myth of the Antidepressant: An Historical Analysis. In: M. Rapley, J. Moncrieff & J. Dillon (Eds.), *De-Medicalising Misery: Psychiatry Psychology and the Human Condition* (pp. 174–188). London: Palgrave Macmillan. https://doi.org/10.1057/9780230342507_13

Moncrieff, J. (2013). *The Bitterest Pills: The Troubling Story of Antipsychotic Drugs*. Basingstoke, Hampshire: Palgrave Macmillan.

Monkey (1978). A TV series created by Wu Cheng'en: Australian Broadcasting Corporation.

Mr Robot (2015). A TV series created by Sam Esmaill: USA Network.

Newman, A. (1995). *Non-Compliance in Winnicott's Words: A Companion to the Work of D.W. Winnicott*. London: Free Association.

Ogden, P., Minton, K., & Pain, C. (2006). *Trauma and the Body: A Sensorimotor Approach to Psychotherapy.* New York: W. W. Norton.

Panksepp, J., & Biven, L. (2012). *The Archaeology of Mind: Neuroevolutionary Origins of Human Emotions.* London: W.W. Norton.

Perel, E. (2007). *Mating in Captivity: Unlocking Erotic Intelligence.* London: Hodder & Stoughton.

Ramirez, N. F. (2016). Why the Baby Brain Can Learn Two Languages at the Same Time. *The Conversation.* [Research scientist at the University of Washington reporting on her research.] https://theconversation.com/why-the-baby-brain-can-learn-two-languages-at-the-same-time-57470

Ransome, A. (1930). *We Didn't Mean to Go to Sea.* London: Jonathan Cape.

Resnick, J. (2016). *How Two Love: Making Your Relationships Work and Last.* Swanbourne, Western Australia: Amygdala.

Sass, L. (1994). *The Paradoxes of Delusion: Wittgenstein, Schreber, and the Schizophrenic Mind.* New York: Cornell.

Schore, A. N. (2012). *The Science of the Art of Psychotherapy.* New York: W. W. Norton.

Schore, A. N. (2015). *Affect Regulation and the Origin of the Self: The Neurobiology of Emotional Development.* Abingdon-on-Thames, Oxfordshire: Routledge.

Schore, A. N. (2019). *Right Brain Psychotherapy.* New York: W. W. Norton.

Shedler, J. (2010). The Efficacy of Psychodynamic Psychotherapy. *American Psychologist, 65*(2): 98–109. https://jonathanshedler.com/PDFs/Shedler%20(2010)%20Efficacy%20of%20Psychodynamic%20Psychotherapy.pdf

Shedler, J. (2017). [adapted from] Where is the Evidence for Evidence-Based Therapy? *Journal of Psychological Therapies in Primary Care, 4*: 47–59 (2015). [The material was originally presented as a keynote address at the Limbus Critical Psychotherapy Conference, Devon, England, 1 November 2014.]   https://jonathanshedler.com/wp-content/uploads/2018/05/Shedler-2018-Where-is-the-evidence-for-evidence-based-therapy.pdf

Siegel, D. (1999). *The Developing Mind: How Relationships and the Brain Interact to Shape Who We Are.* New York: Guilford.

Spitzer, R. L. (1980). Introduction. In: *Diagnostic and Statistical Manual of Mental Disorders Third Edition.* Washington, DC: American Psychiatric Association.

Stern, D. B. (2003). *Unformulated Experience: From Dissociation to Imagination in Psychoanalysis.* Hillsdale, NJ: The Analytic Press.

Stern, D. B. (2010). *Partners in Thought, Working with Unformulated Experience, Dissociation, and Enactment.* New York: Routledge.

Stern, D. B. (2019). *The Infinity of the Unsaid: Unformulated Experience, Language, and the Nonverbal.* New York: Routledge.

Stern, D. N. (1998). *The Motherhood Constellation: A Unified View of Parent-Infant Psychotherapy.* Abingdon-on-Thames: Routledge.

Szasz, T. (1990). *The Untamed Tongue: A Dissenting Dictionary.* La Salle, IL: Open Court.

Tavernise, S. (2016, 22 April). U.S. Suicide Rate Surges to a 30-Year High. *New York Times.* http://www.nytimes.com/2016/04/22/health/us-suicide-rate-surges-to-a-30-year-high.html?_r=0

The American Psychological Association (2012). *Recognition of Psychotherapy Effectiveness.* https://www.apa.org/about/policy/resolution-psychotherapy

The Stepford Wives (1975). Directed by Bryan Forbes. Columbia Pictures Films.

van der Kolk, B. A. (2104). *The Body Keeps the Score: Brain, Mind and Body in the Healing of Trauma.* New York: Viking.

Vaughan, S. C. (2019). *The Talking Cure: The Science Behind Psychotherapy.* International Psychotherapy Institute (ebook). www.freepsychotherapybooks.org

Winnicott, D. W. (1958). *Through Paediatrics to Psychoanalysis.* London: Hogarth.

Winnicott, D. W. (1971). *Playing and Reality.* London: Tavistock.

Yong, E. (2019). A Waste of 1,000 Research Papers—Decades of Early Research on the Genetics of Depression were Built on Non-Existent Foundations. How Did That Happen? *The Atlantic*, 17 May. https://www.theatlantic.com/science/archive/2019/05/waste-1000-studies/589684/

Wittgenstein, L. (1953). *Philosophical Investigations.* Basingstoke, Hampshire: Macmillan.

About the author

Jan lives with his wife Cath in Perth, Western Australia, and has six children and three grandchildren. His practice is Amygdala Consulting where he consults in psychoanalytic psychotherapy and offers clinical supervision. He has practised for over forty-five years. He trained in London where he was supervised by R. D. Laing, John M. Heaton, and Christopher Bollas. He moved to Australia in 1990 where he founded The Churchill Clinic that ran nationally accredited professional trainings. The founding president of the Psychotherapists & Counsellors Association of Western Australia, Jan received an Outstanding Achievement award for his contribution to the profession. He was an Editorial Advisory Board member of the national journal *Psychotherapy in Australia*, where he penned a regular column for over twenty years. An Advisory Board member of Blue Knot Foundation (formerly Adult Survivors of Child Abuse), Jan is also an accredited supervisor for the Royal Australian/New Zealand College of Psychiatrists in psychotherapy and supervises Developmental Paediatricians at the State Child Development Centre (West Perth).

Jan Resnick has a PhD in Psychology (psychoanalysis) based on a psychotherapeutic understanding and treatment of psychosomatic disorders. Over his career, he founded and presided over four separate mental health charities. He has over one hundred publishing credits including his first published book *How Two Love: Making Your Relationship Work and Last* (2016) based on his clinical work with couples.

He still plays piano and basketball and remains an avid football fan.

Index